FRANK SEPE'S
ABS-OLUTELY
PERFECT PLAN FOR A
FLATTER STOMACH

ALSO BY FRANK SEPE

*The **TRUTH:** The <u>Only</u> Fitness Book You'll Ever Need*

———

HAY HOUSE TITLES OF RELATED INTEREST

Books

BodyChange™: *The 21-Day Fitness Program for Changing Your Body . . . and Changing Your Life!* by Montel Williams and Wini Linguvic

Every Move You Make: *Bodymind Exercises to Transform Your Life,* by Nikki Winston

Shape® Magazine's Shape Your Life: *4 Weeks to a Better Body—and a Better Life,* by Barbara Harris, editor-in-chief, *Shape* magazine, with Angela Hynes

Ultimate Pilates, by Dreas Reyneke

Yoga Pure and Simple, by Kisen

Kits

8 Minutes in the Morning® Kit:
A Simple Way to Shed Up to 2 Pounds a Week—Guaranteed, by Jorge Cruise

8 Minutes in the Morning® to a Flat Belly Kit:
Lose Up to 6 Inches in Less than 4 Weeks—Guaranteed, by Jorge Cruise

———

All of the above are available at your local bookstore, or may be ordered by visiting:
Hay House USA: **www.hayhouse.com**
Hay House Australia: **www.hayhouse.com.au**
Hay House UK: **www.hayhouse.co.uk**
Hay House South Africa: **orders@psdprom.co.za**

FRANK SEPE'S
ABS-OLUTELY
PERFECT PLAN FOR A
FLATTER STOMACH

THE *ONLY* ABS BOOK YOU'LL EVER NEED!

FRANK SEPE

HAY HOUSE, INC.
Carlsbad, California
London • Sydney • Johannesburg
Vancouver • Hong Kong

Published and distributed in the United States by: Hay House, Inc., P.O. Box 5100, Carlsbad, CA 92018-5100 • *Phone:* (760) 431-7695 or (800) 654-5126 • *Fax:* (760) 431-6948 or (800) 650-5115 • www.hayhouse.com • **Published and distributed in Australia by:** Hay House Australia Pty. Ltd., 18/36 Ralph St., Alexandria NSW 2015 • *Phone:* 612-9669-4299 • *Fax:* 612-9669-4144 • www.hayhouse.com.au • **Published and distributed in the United Kingdom by:** Hay House UK, Ltd. • Unit 62, Canalot Studios • 222 Kensal Rd., London W10 5BN • *Phone:* 44-20-8962-1230 • *Fax:* 44-20-8962-1239 • www.hayhouse.co.uk • **Published and distributed in the Republic of South Africa by:** Hay House SA (Pty), Ltd., P.O. Box 990, Witkoppen 2068 • *Phone/Fax:* 2711-7012233 • orders@psdprom.co.za • **Distributed in Canada by:** Raincoast • 9050 Shaughnessy St., Vancouver, B.C. V6P 6E5 • *Phone:* (604) 323-7100 • *Fax:* (604) 323-2600

Editorial supervision: Jill Kramer
Design: Summer McStravick
Interior photos: Sean Kahlil, with the exception of those on pages vi, 3, 195, and 196 (PhotoDisc) and on pages xix, 53, 69, 149, and 159 (BananaStock).

Library of Congress Cataloging-in-Publication Data

Sepe, Frank, 1971-
Frank Sepe's abs-olutely perfect plan for a flatter stomach : the only abs book you'll ever need / Frank Sepe.
     p. cm.
ISBN 1-4019-0527-7 (hardcover)
1. Abdominal exercises. 2. Physical fitness. I. Title.
GV508.S46 2005
613.7'1—dc22

2004014443

ISBN 1-4019-0527-7

08 07 06 05   4 3 2 1
1st printing, January 2005

Printed in China through Palace Press International

Contents

(**Author's Note:** Always consult your physician or other health-care provider before beginning any exercise, nutritional, or weight-loss program, especially if you suffer from a bad back, heart disease, or other medical problem or condition. If you're going to engage in weight-training exercise, I strongly recommend that you consult with a licensed fitness trainer or expert.)

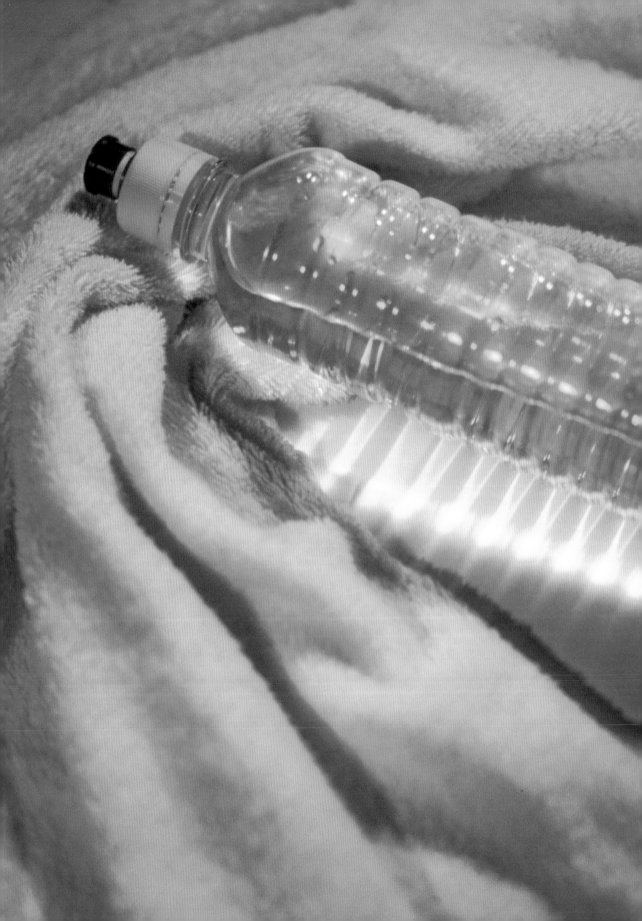

Foreword

It's an understatement to say that I was a bit surprised when Frank asked me to write the Foreword for his new book. Perhaps his reason was that in some circles, people see me as a celebrity. Now, Frank is actually a man who's "in the know." He's also connected to celebrities who are far more famous in every sense of the word than I am—I mean, the guy tones up models, sports heroes, and TV and movie stars.

So . . . why me? Sure, I've come to know Frank very well, and have learned that wit and sarcasm are as much of his personality as is his drive for teaching people how to achieve the body of their dreams. But let's forget about the body parts for a second and ask again: Why me?

I'm still not so sure. In fact, a few months ago, I'd come to the conclusion that Frank was kidding when he asked me to write this! I actually didn't give it another thought until the morning he reminded me that I'd need to submit my Foreword to him as soon as possible because the book was going to print in a few months.

There was only one thing to do: Panic. Then I thought, *Wow—he's serious! And I don't even have washboard abs!*

When I realized that Frank was waiting for my copy, I finally turned to him one morning during my workout session, wiped some sweat off my brow, and asked, "Frank, why me?"

His response was typical of what anyone lucky enough to know him in person (and I'm happy to call him a friend after working out with him for more than a year) finds out: "You *get* it," he said.

I didn't have to read anything into those three words, and I certainly didn't question what he meant.

More than a year ago, I was getting a little chunky. My scale logged in at 200 pounds. As much as I'd love to tell you the age-old excuse that "most of it was muscle," of course, it wasn't. It was just plain ol' fat. Making matters worse, I was on a lecture tour, and everywhere I went, the local stations happened to be playing much older episodes of the TV show I host called

Crossing Over. It's not that I have a problem watching myself on the small screen—but I do have a problem watching my *significantly thinner* self.

I was in that place that I'm sure many of you reading this are in now: I wasn't happy with my body. So, on a very long flight back from Australia, I was complaining to Reid Tracy, the president of Hay House (and my publisher) that I needed to find a trainer and take my workouts much more seriously. He suggested that I work out with their top fitness author, a guy by the name of Frank Sepe. Reid went on to explain that the company was just getting ready to release Frank's first book on dieting and exercise. Making this story even better was when he casually told me, "Frank even lives near you in Long Island."

Since my publisher is from California, I silently laughed at that last one because I knew Long Island is a very big place. Nevertheless, Reid gave me Frank's number, and as a favor to our mutual publisher, Frank agreed to meet with me. Luckily, we hit it off (and we *did* live near each other). Ever since that first meeting, Frank has been educating me when it comes to the world of fitness and nutrition.

I hope he never stops.

THESE DAYS, FRANK WILL LOOK AT ME and repeat, "You get it." What I get is that there's no magic pill or quick fix to accomplish your fitness goals. Nothing beats time and commitment when it comes to making permanent changes to your overall physical health.

I remember the day Frank asked, "John, what do you want to achieve with me?"

Without hesitation, I said, "Abs—I want a six-pack. I ordered them for my 30th birthday, but apparently they're on back order at the warehouse, so maybe we need a new plan."

Frank laughed and quickly retorted, "You can't spot-reduce. Lesson one." Then he told me that I needed to mentally enroll myself in a three-step program: weight resistance, cardio training, and (yes) diet. That was what my situation boiled down to. Or as he says, "That's the truth."

After following Frank's regimen (which he wrote about in great detail in his first book, *The TRUTH*), I'm happy to report today that I've lost more than 15 pounds, have dropped my cholesterol level, and have given up my membership in the "yo-yo dieting club" of low-fat, low-carb, high-protein, no-joy meals. Now I follow a nutritional plan that doesn't make me think I'm starving.

But back to my six-pack. . . . Frank and I are at a point in my program where the dream of great abs isn't just a dream anymore—it's a reality. It's still about sweat, though, because there's no pill, video, magic exercise machine, or tasty juice from a tree in Bora-Bora that will give me those coveted abs. (Darn!) All I truly need in order to get them is knowledge. And that's what you're going to find in this book. You'll see how to get your own six-pack—or whatever type of abs you desire.

Now, many of you are probably thinking that I have an advantage over you because Frank Sepe is my personal trainer. You're right! But I also know that after reading this book and following his principles, you'll have Frank as *your* trainer as well. And then, you'll get it, too.

WITHIN THESE PAGES, you'll find a selection of exercises coupled with Frank's experience in fitness and nutrition, which has made him one of the most photographed fitness cover models in the world. You'll read about the idea of "mixing it up" and changing your program around. Frank gives you options so that you don't feel as if you're doing the same boring routine day after day. That really does make a difference.

As for me, I'm with the program, but I'm not Frank's best client. Unfortunately, I don't jump out of bed in the morning and think, *I can't wait to eat well and exercise today! Bring it on!* Please don't tell Frank, but I'd much rather eat chocolate cake and guzzle soda. (And that's just my dream breakfast!) I'd also love it if I never had to look at another piece of cardio equipment ever again.

But just like you, that reality isn't possible for me any longer. So when I'm feeling lazy, I try to remind myself of how just a few years ago it was deemed "cool" and even socially acceptable to smoke. Today, we know that it kills. I also know now that eating more nutritiously and working out isn't an option, it's a necessity. I hate to admit it, but it isn't just about getting those washboard abs—it's about being healthy.

I wish all of you the best on your own personal quest to become fit human beings. Good luck finding the true you. And let me remind you of three little words that Frank uses on me for motivation. (Or are they a warning?)

"Drop the cookie!" he insists.

It's good advice.

— **John Edward,** June 2004

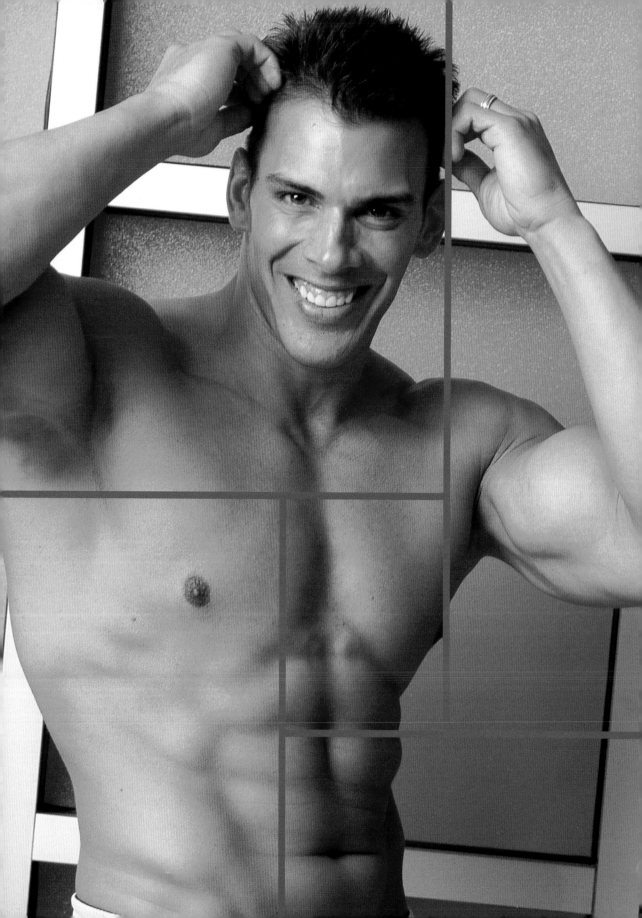

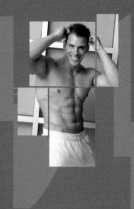

INTRODUCTION

WHO IS FRANK SEPE, AND WHAT THE HECK DOES HE KNOW ABOUT ABS?

There are few absolutes in this life, but some of my personal favorites include: Chicken soup actually does make you feel better; your mother really does know best; and we'd be a much healthier nation if we all just dropped the cookie—but more on this one a few chapters down the road.

Oh, my favorite absolute in life takes me back to my own childhood in New York City. I'm sorry that this isn't going to be one of those joyful memories because I'm taking you back to my sixth-grade playground at P.S. 138 Middle School in Rosedale, Queens.

I was a skinny kid with a big mouth, but my loose lips were no match for the big bullies by the monkey bars. They'd shove me around just for the heck of it, and then they'd unload the most vicious childhood taunt in the book: "Sepe, we hate your guts!"

Looking at my six-pack stomach these days, I don't think that line would still ring true today. In fact, I saw some of those bullies (now in their 30s) the other day hanging around the old neighborhood. One of them even came up to me—but this time, he didn't greet me with a shove; instead, he gave me a look of amazement as he unwrapped a king-sized Snickers bar. "Yo, Frank, do ya think if I did a few sit-ups, I could look like you?" he asked.

Here's comes another absolute: No, a few sit-ups won't do the trick—but if this guy followed my program over time, we could take the mountain out of the middle of this man.

Anyone can have great abs, which is my way of saying, "Hello. Thank you for picking up my book." The minute you opened it, you added one more absolute to your life: *You don't have to hate your own guts anymore.*

It's just that simple.

LET'S BEGIN WITH A LITTLE AUDIENCE PARTICIPATION. Put this book down for a second and really look at your stomach. I know that about 90 percent of you out there aren't too happy right now. Well, the good news is that your abs won't be looking this way for much longer—you're about to give them a huge kiss-off. This program will change your midsection from "flab to fab." So let's get started.

The first step doesn't include one crunch or even getting out a mat. I promise that you won't feel sore tomorrow if you do one little thing for me right now, and it's one of the most important when it comes to my program. Before you read another word, you must admit to yourself that it's time to make a change. You have to be able to make a 100 percent commitment, both mentally and physically to this (or any other) plan. If you don't take that key first step, then you're destined for failure.

Congratulations—you're still with me! That means you've made the commitment.

For those of you who haven't read my first book, *The TRUTH: The Only Fitness Book You'll Ever Need,* what are you waiting for? (Just kidding.) Seriously, that book contains everything you need to know for making positive mental and physical changes in your body. I prefer to think of it as a step-by-step plan in which the end result is wellness.

If you haven't had the chance to pick up that book yet, then you may be wondering just who you're committing the next several weeks to in order to achieve a better body. In other words, *Who is Frank Sepe, and what does he know about abs?*

Well, I'm someone who embraced fitness as a way of life as a teenager. I also get extreme joy out of educating people and making positive changes in their lives. I'm not your typical fitness expert or whatever term people use these days. I like to joke that we should be called "super trainers," like "supermodels." But I digress . . . if you see me on the street, I prefer Frank.

I'm different from other fitness professionals in that I live, practice, and preach what I write in my books. I'm the guy who knows (from a lifetime of fitness study and applications) how to help you achieve and maintain a fantastic body. I'm a former champion bodybuilder who's been training for 20 years, and educating people on health and fitness for the past decade. I'm the author of the aforementioned best-selling book, *The TRUTH,* and I'm an editor and monthly columnist for *American Health & Fitness Magazine* and *MuscleMag International.*

As a fitness trainer, I've worked with celebrities, athletes, and everyday Joes and Josephines. I'm also a spokesperson for MET-Rx and have conducted dozens of seminars on the body. You might also know me as a model who's appeared on hundreds of magazine covers. I should also mention that I'm the fitness expert on ESPN2's show *Cold Pizza.*

In other words, I've been in this business long enough to know my stuff, and I also take great pride in what I do. I've personally done the ab routines in this book for the past 20 years, and I know they work—and not only for me, but for thousands of others. All my routines have been battle tested and have made a positive difference in the lives of people who've made them a part of their fitness regimen.

Over the past ten years, I've built a solid reputation as a trainer. But it's not enough that I give myself that job title—I'm someone who gets results. After all, the last thing I want is for my clients to spend the time and energy on a program that only works halfway. It's all or nothing for me: I don't just want results; I want *incredible* results.

Take a look at my photo on the cover. It's not some secret how I got to look this way—it's not voodoo or an ancient blessing (I wish). It's the same hard work that we'll do together in this book.

As for my own abs, well, they're a little bit famous. So far, they don't have an attitude, but you never know. My abs want you to know that they've been profiled in about 100 magazines.

My body is my business, and fitness is my life. You can bet that I won't make you feel the burn of another program that doesn't work.

WHEN I WAS A LITTLE KID, my father told me, "Son, find a job you love to do, and you'll be good at it." When I was 13, I followed my wise dad's advice . . . only I didn't know it.

I started weight training to strengthen my skinny body. At first it was just a way to defend myself from getting the crud kicked out of me every day at school, but then I just knew it was for me. It was thrilling to watch my body change, and even better were all those compliments I started getting from girls who wanted to touch my biceps. Yes, I loved being the center of attention, but I really loved challenging my body to reach the next level.

One day, I took off my Pac-Man T-shirt and realized that I was looking pretty good. I didn't exactly have defined abs, but at least the ones peeking out weren't covered with flab. And, even better, I wasn't a bag of bones anymore.

I'll never forget that first post-training moment I hit Jones Beach in Long Island with my teenage friends. Imagine a typical New York summer day, where it's 95 degrees in the shade with 100 percent humidity. The guys in my posse had planned to meet up with a group of girls, which was quite serious business. It also required a high level of planning and discussion on the way to the beach.

"Who do you think you'll hook up with?" I asked my buddy Billy as we walked the steaming hot mile from the parking lot to the beach.

Billy started describing a cute blonde from geometry class. I wasn't really listening to him because my mind was filled with important thoughts: *I've been working out like crazy. These girls are going to love my body—they won't be able to take their eyes off me! I bet there might even be a fight for who's going to hang with me all day.*

When we got to the beach and met up with actual bikini-wearing girls, I thought I'd finally arrived at a land we'll call "Young Man's Heaven." Immediately, Sally, a gorgeous redhead from biology class, walked up to us, and in the sweetest voice I've ever heard said, "Oh my God! Look at that guy's body! It's awesome." (By the way, *awesome* was just about the best thing you could hear back in those days. It was cooler than *cool*.)

Naturally, I couldn't contain my smile because Sally had such great taste, and what a nice girl—she was so free with the compliments! I was ready to make my move when it dawned on me that we weren't making any sort of eye contact. In fact, Sally was staring over my shoulder toward a buff dude who was leaning against his red Corvette.

"That guy," Sally said, pointing to Mr. Awesome Car, "has the best abs I've ever seen in my life!"

Turning around in disgust, I gave the guy another glance, and I had to admit that he was living the dream. Not only did he possess those great wheels, but he also had what we now call a shredded six-pack stomach.

They call these moments an epiphany. I realized that I was spending all this time training to get my arms and chest bigger, and I'd completely missed the point: I had to work on building the best-looking *total* physique. And nine times out of ten, when people refer to someone as having "a hot body," it has a lot to do with their midsection.

Back on the beach, I realized that my body was incomplete. So, walking that mile to the car in the heat and humidity, I made the decision to start training my abs. I knew that that was the only way to have the type of body that got the stares. (Oh, and by the way, I never did get a date with Sally. If she's still with Six-Pack Guy, I hope they're happy and she gets to drive that car if he still owns it.)

When I got home that day, I shook the sand out of my shoes and began to read everything I could find on the subject of abdominals. Unfortunately, it was the 1980s, so I couldn't just go home and Google "abs." Back then, you had two choices: You either had to buy a Jane Fonda workout tape or head to the newsstand.

As a tough guy, I ditched Jane for the magazine rack, but there weren't 200 different monthly glossies on the market at that time. However, I did pick up a stray muscle mag because I was already a huge collector of them. I went back through my archives and ripped out every article on abs I could find. I'd skipped over these stories in the past, but now they became like a bible to me.

I've always thought that before you train, it helps to work out your mind. Information is key to any program. To that end, I memorized every ab routine in those magazines and decided to follow the route of pro bodybuilders because they basically have the best abs in the entire world. *If I just do what they do, I'll be back on the beach with Sally checking <u>me</u> out in no time,* I decided.

It sounded like a good idea, but unfortunately the results weren't so hot. Instead of start- ing small, I followed the plan of the three-time Mr. Universe. (Hey, why not try to start at the top?) Just thinking about this makes my stomach ache, even though it's many years later. To put it sim- ply, the routine was absolutely insane. But I thought, *If it's in a magazine and someone printed it and the guy looks pretty good, then it's my solution, too.* I knew that if I just put in the sweat and time, I'd look like a three-time Mr. Universe as well.

The routine called for a daily total of 25 sets of abs. Think about that for a minute—we're talking *25 sets!* In other words, this guy did 15–25 reps *of each set.* Now, even a seasoned veteran who's been training his abs for ten years knows that this routine is a one-way ticket to destroying the stomach. You can just imagine the impact it had on a 16-year-old kid who was gung ho and wanted to impress the chicks. I put everything into my 25 daily sets, finishing each routine even if my abs were screaming in pain. I thought that if it almost killed me, then it must be making me stronger.

Big mistake—these routines almost *did* kill me. I'd crunch away until one day I couldn't stand up straight. I tried to walk upstairs, but I couldn't move. It felt as if someone had hit me in the stomach with a sledgehammer. Finally hobbling upstairs a few minutes later, I went to bed in pure agony. Luckily, I fell asleep in my misery only to wake up a few hours later with an unusual problem. I couldn't lift myself out of the bed. Since it's abs that help us lift ourselves off the comfy mattress each morning, I was in a world of hurt. And even after my mother assisted me out of bed, I still couldn't stand up straight. At school that day, my abs kept suddenly cramping as if someone had reached inside me to squeeze my muscles in the cruelest and hardest way possible.

That was my first experience with ab exercises, thank you very much.

I could have easily quit after that, but fortunately my desire to achieve my fitness goals made me persevere, although not right away. First I had to heal, which took about two weeks. When I felt better, I looked through my magazines and found a different routine that wasn't so difficult. I started doing these exercises almost every single day.

I must have tried every conceivable abdominal routine from the age of 16 to 19. It was pure luck that I began to form anything resembling a toned midsection back then, and I credit three different life forces for helping me along because my regimen wasn't so hot: (1) I had a fast metabolism, which meant that my body-fat percentage was low—this is key for great abs; (2) I was blessed with good genes, which meant that I was a naturally thin person (please don't hate me); and (3) I was going through good old puberty—I just kept getting taller, so any weight I did put on was evenly distributed on my body.

However, my actions weren't helping out my three gifts. Yes, I was training my abs, but I kept eating the major teenage food groups, including potato chips, soda, pizza, and my personal favorite, chicken pot pie. Is there anything better on this planet, except perhaps consuming all those things in one day? (By the way, we won't be doing that in this book. Sorry I had to break it to you. . . .)

My views on dieting were a bit different in the 1980s. I was clueless to the fact that what I was eating had a huge effect on the development of my body—or, should I say, the *lack* of development, even though I was working out on a regular basis. I'd decided that the more I ate the better, because I knew I'd just pack on the weight, work out, and then turn that mass into ripped muscle. It's not that I was an idiot; it's just that the magazines I read never printed stories about eating right—they just said to hit the exercise mat.

Back then I believed what a lot of people still do today, which is that you just have to train to get great abs. If it were that easy, I'd be eating a bag of Fritos right now.

No, great abs begin with cleaning up your eating habits. There's no way around that one.

AT AGE 19, I STARTED TRAINING WITH LARRY PEPE, a professional bodybuilder who changed my views on nutrition forever. There I was, pumping iron at my local gym, when Larry and I started to talk about bodybuilding. When he asked if I'd like to help him out with his upcoming competition, I jumped at the chance. That's when I began to learn what it really took to get the body in maximum shape.

Larry would even talk to me about nutrition. "What did you eat yesterday, Frank?" he'd demand. "I want you to give me the complete list of foods you put into your body."

"Uh . . . three chicken pot pies, two slices of pizza, five Cokes, and a Hershey bar—but I only had a few bites of it," I stammered.

I can still see my new friend clutching his heart when he heard this menu plan. "Thank God you're young," he said. "If you were any older, you'd be pushing 300 pounds."

Larry began to explain to me the kinds of foods I should be eating if I wanted to have the best physique possible. Ever the nice guy, he even took the time to put together a diet program for me. Meanwhile, we trained together for the next ten weeks as he prepared for his bodybuilding competition. During that time, something amazing happened to my body: I went from one extreme to the other. Remember my abs of nothing? Well, now they had some definition.

I like the expression "Seeing is believing." In my case, I couldn't quite believe what I was seeing. In fact, my entire body was reaching a new fitness level and acquiring a lean, cut, sculpted shape. You see, it wasn't just the exercises that were causing this shift. For the first time in my life, I was eating correctly while doing cardiovascular exercises, in addition to working out with weights. The combination of the three components changed my life forever—as it will yours if you follow my plan.

Let's sum it up now: I had a new physique. Physically, I felt so strong that I could have moved a building, while mentally, I was on top of the world. Of course, I was inspired to keep pushing my body to the maximum. As you'll see for yourself when you do the exercises in this book, a few minor physical changes will push you toward greater glory. Be sure to reward yourself for the small victories because they'll keep you motivated and shove you in the direction of wanting more for yourself. After all, it's when we become complacent and unmotivated that we fall into a negative tailspin that keeps us from achieving any of our goals.

One quick note: I can't lie to you and say that from that point on, I became an eating purist. My life didn't solely revolve around grilled chicken and lettuce. We all have our good eating days and our not-so-hot, pass-the-grease, another-helping-of-sugar days. I mean, I've had more than a few bad meals in my life, and over the years, I've opened the door to my local pizza parlor quite a bit. I shouldn't admit it, but the owner actually knows me by name. Nevertheless, I can say that my good nutrition days definitely outnumber my bad ones by a huge margin.

Slowly but surely, abs became my gateway to a better body. I know that sounds weird to say, but once I achieved my six-pack, many doors opened for me—for example, I became a successful model and began participating in bodybuilding competitions. Oh, and great-looking women also started to go out with me. Okay, that last one is just a joke, but I did get a few dates. Maybe it was my personality; maybe it was my abs. It certainly wasn't my budget back then (hence, all those pizza stops).

Now, WHAT ABOUT *YOUR* MIDSECTION? You should know right away that my *ABS-olutely Perfect Plan for a Flatter Stomach* isn't a quick-fix program. It doesn't promise unrealistic and unattainable results in no time flat. It isn't going to give you a rock-hard midriff in three minutes a day. It's not going to help you lose 100 pounds in two weeks. You're not going to become a runway model or a Chippendales dancer by this time next week. In other words, I refuse to give you promises I can't keep.

This book *will* give you all the information you need to take your entire body—not just your abs—to a new and improved level. During this process, I'll tell you which exercises are the best, and I'll explain specific routines that will achieve the best results. We'll also cover what you should eat and how much cardio you need to do.

All your questions on how to achieve the best possible midsection will be answered in this book, which I've broken down into three different sections: The first will give you a quick education when it comes to your abs; the second discusses important factors that will make you succeed or fail, including nutrition and cardio; and the third will feature the 15 ab exercises you can do absolutely anywhere.

Ready for your first lesson?

Drop the cookie.

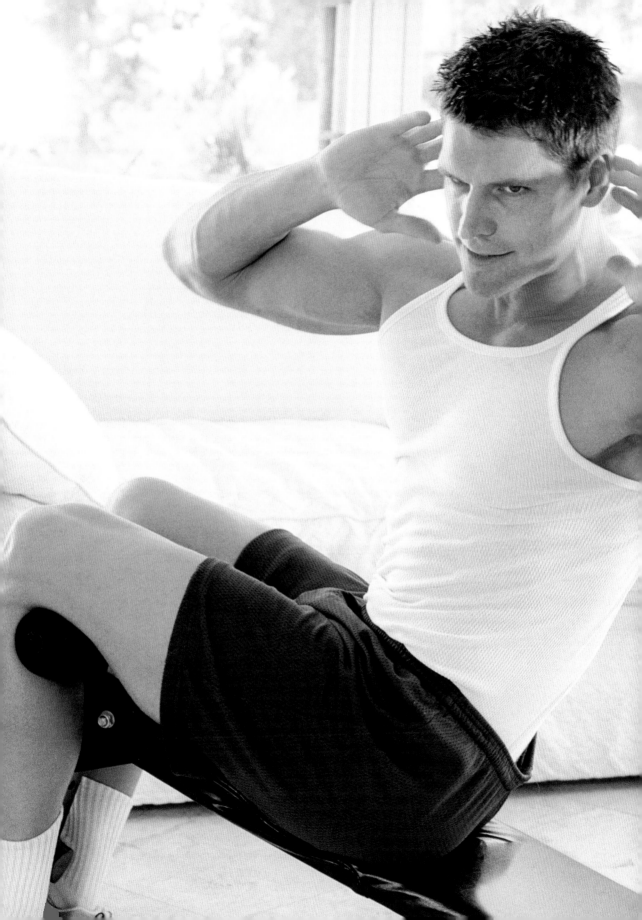

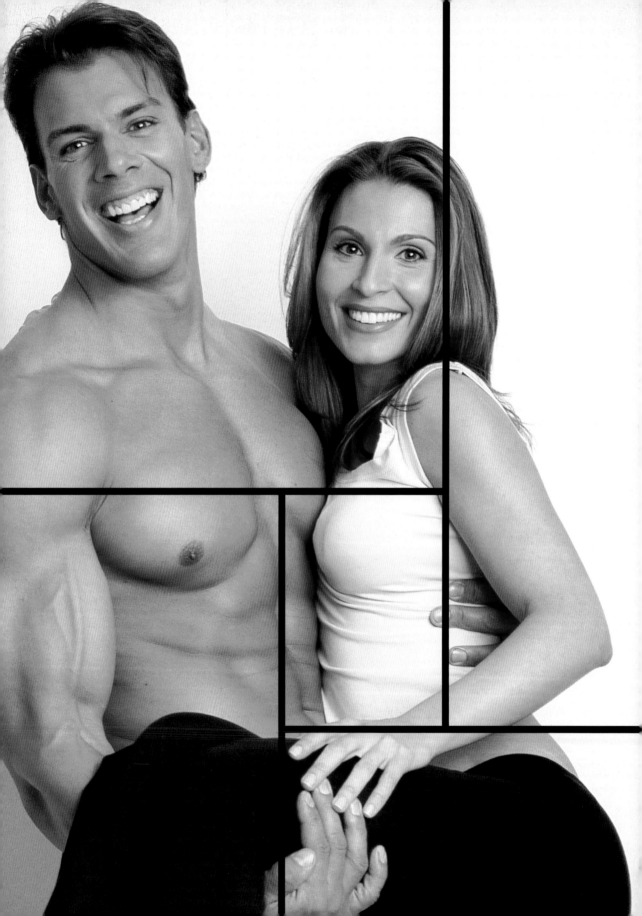

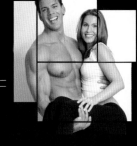

PART I

An ABS-olute Ab Education

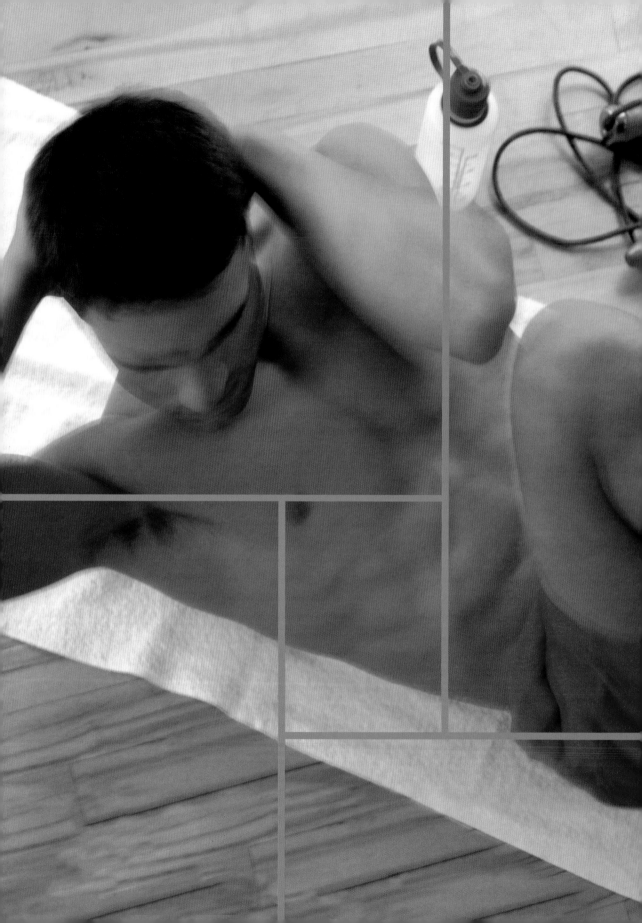

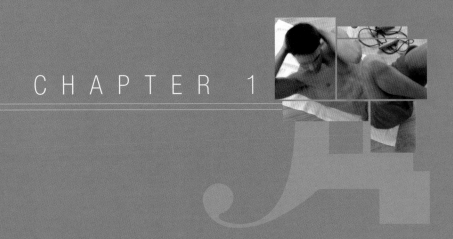

ABS-OLUTE AB PITFALLS

It's Saturday afternoon and you're channel surfing . . . when you see that ab machine infomercial. Of course it's hard not to stop and watch, because there's a very toned man promising that if you buy his contraption for three easy payments of $99.99 plus shipping and handling, you can acquire a six-pack in no time flat. Suddenly you're thinking, *Wow, that seems easy . . . I like easy! I can just get on this flimsy-looking machine for 5 or 10 minutes a day and have the abs of my dreams!*

If that scenario sounds familiar to you, take comfort. I have friends who have actually shelled out the cash for one of these dream machines, which they tend to use for about a week. When it becomes apparent that this gadget won't be the answer to their prayers, it finds a new life as the most expensive coatrack in the house. That's when I get the blistering phone call: "Frank, why didn't this work? They promised me! Plus, I still have to make two payments."

"Go back and tape the infomercial," I say. "Pause when you get to the teeny-tiny writing on the bottom of the screen that says, 'The machine works when used in conjunction with a diet-and-exercise regimen.'"

Clearly, those machines don't constitute a total-body program by themselves. I'll go into more depth on this topic in a later chapter, but please don't feel bad if you're also the proud owner of a new coatrack. It's really great for hanging up dress pants before you pack for a big trip. Seriously, these machines are useful as a part of a complete fitness plan. There are even some pretty good ones out there. But alone, they're not the solution.

In this chapter, we'll look at some other obstacles that could be blocking you from possessing the abs of your dreams.

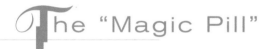 The "Magic Pill"

You should be wary of any program that promises you unbelievable results by just popping a pill. *You won't turn into a Greek god or goddess by using anything that comes out of a bottle.* Taking a pill without exercising and following a solid nutritional plan will *never* get you the benefits you want. You have a better chance of striking oil in your backyard than building a six-pack with a pill.

You only get results from hard work and a good, solid plan. After all, if you could get toned abs from a bottle, then the manufacturer would be the richest person on Earth. Sure, supplements can help, but you need to check with your doctor first and read the labels carefully. There's no reason to put yourself at risk by taking harmful ingredients.

A lot of people go to the health-food store and just grab a bottle off the shelf without noting the ingredients—they simply read what the pill's supposed to do. News flash: A lot of these drugs aren't approved by the FDA and can cause extreme damage to your body. I can't stress enough how important it is to become label savvy. Research the ingredients and know what you're taking. Ask yourself a few questions: What exactly does this pill do? What are the side effects? What happens if you take it in conjunction with other drugs?

Some common diet pills on the market contain ingredients including caffeine, creatine, synephrine, and hydroxy methylbutyrate (or HMB). Some of you may have been taking these products for years without any problems; while for others, one or two pills can be detrimental. The reason for this disparity is that many of us don't know if we have heart or liver problems until we start feeling symptoms. So if you have high blood pressure and you start taking diet products that contain enormous amounts of caffeine, synephrine, or green-tea extract, you could land in intensive care.

Remember that it wasn't so long ago that thousands of stores across the country were peddling ephedrine . . . until people started complaining of adverse side effects. When two high-profile professional athletes died, their sudden demises were blamed on the use of ephedrine-based items. Whether or not this was in fact true, the government subsequently issued a ban on all such products.

Why even put yourself at risk? Is the lure of getting a six-pack by just popping a pill that tempting? Be smart and sensible.

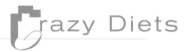

Crazy Diets

If I gave you a diet that consisted of 40 grapes a day, you'd lose weight. If I told you to eat one hamburger and some fries a day, you'd lose some weight. The same goes for eating one candy bar and 12 glasses of water a day. I know that most of the eating plans out there don't sound this far-fetched, but go do some research. I bet you'll find diets similar to the wacky ones I've outlined above.

Here's the truth about crazy diet plans: Since they all restrict your calories, you'll lose weight in the short term. In fact, you might even drop four or five pounds in the first week. You'll think, *Wow, this is the solution!* Wrong. Basically, you're shedding water and losing muscle, especially if you're not consuming enough protein. You'll also notice that you have no energy to work out if the diet doesn't contain enough carbohydrates and fats. And then there's the danger of slowing down your metabolism and gaining even more weight when you ditch the insane program.

An eating plan isn't just about losing weight; rather, it's supposed to help you maintain and build lean muscle mass; give you energy; and create a happier, healthier you. Fad diets don't do any of that good stuff. They make you unhealthy, give you a dismal outlook mentally when it comes to taking care of your body, and cause you to feel like a failure because you can't stay on track. Who could? How can anyone get through the day when they constantly feel so hungry and tired? These diets make you feel miserable, and in turn, you're probably making everyone around you feel the same way.

It all goes back to embracing the idea of getting in shape as a lifestyle. You need to exercise and follow a sensible eating program for your *entire life.* And that's the only way you're going to be able to achieve and maintain a flat, good-looking midsection, too.

Keep in mind that fad diets are harmful, short-term fixes—they won't give you a foundation to build on that will help you achieve your goals.

Unrealistic Expectations

Now let's look at the advertising industry for a second, beginning with the most common way they hook us with these body-beautiful products. It begins with the seemingly perfect model who's hawking the item—you want to look like that person, which is understandable. But every time you're tempted to fall into this trap, please remember one thing: These models have dieted and trained *for years* to achieve those fantastic abs. You're seeing them in their best shape. After all, this is their job.

Take it from an ab model—I'd never do a photo shoot unless my midsection was in top form. How I look is based on training, dieting, genetics, photography, camera angles, correct lighting, flexing, oil that's smeared on my abs, makeup, and so on. All these elements come into play when I'm hired to sell a product. Now when you, the consumer, just glance at an image, remember what goes into developing that picture-perfect look! If you buy these products, you won't immediately look like the model . . . in fact, you might *never* look like him or her.

Along the same lines, it drives me crazy to see all those "before and after" ad campaigns. Now, don't get me wrong: Some of these folks have legitimately worked hard to become an "after," and I applaud anyone who achieves any goal. However, there are many people in these ads who are totally bogus. Think about the individual who claims he lost 50 pounds in six weeks by using a tiny machine for two minutes a day. Notice the "after" photo: He looks thinner, taller, and perhaps his face is even different. That's because many of these photos are doctored by computers to achieve such a radical transformation.

The bigger question to ask yourself is: "Does this make sense?" That is, could *anyone* lose 50 pounds in six weeks from two minutes a day of effort? I think you know the answer.

These ads feed our expectations because we *want* to look and feel our best. The desire to get there clouds our decision-making process. Realize that you're being duped, and read between the lines—don't believe these ads. Also, don't compete against these models; compete against yourself.

You're not a failure if you don't look like a model. You're simply improving your own body to become the best, healthiest you possible. And to me, that makes you a successful person.

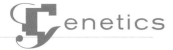enetics

Everyone has abs, but what kind? Well, the first step is to know that your stomach muscles are covered with fat—once you get rid of it, the clearer the muscles can be seen. Some people will find that when they remove the fat, they have a six-pack, while others will see a four-pack. I even knew a guy who was the proud owner of an eight-pack.

You can thank your mother and father if you get those perfect washboard abs, but don't blame them if you don't. Remember that everyone's middle looks much better when the fat is gone. I know several Victoria's Secret models who aren't moaning that they don't have a six-pack. They have beautiful bodies and live with the fact that they're just a certain way genetically. And some of the greatest bodybuilders in the world have a four-pack. The point is that genetics determines what you'll end up revealing—you can't change your DNA, but you *can* define what God gave you.

Also keep in mind that everyone has a different genetic makeup, and this is what will determine how fast you'll acquire toned abs, and what they'll look like when you get them. Let's say that you follow the exact same program as a friend. You may or may not advance as fast as this person because some people just have a genetic propensity toward exercise, which makes them progress at a much faster rate. So please don't get caught up in creating the most perfect midsection in the world—just make the best of the one you were given. Believe me, it will be more than good enough.

pot-Reduction

The notion of "spot-reduction" is the biggest myth going in fitness. Listen carefully when I tell you that it's impossible to pick a particular area of the body to tone. The body loses weight systematically and holistically, not one part at a time.

Your genes do determine where your body fat is stored. However, you can't just work on "trouble areas"—all you end up doing is developing stronger muscles underneath the stored fat. Genetics will determine where the fat comes off first. Generally, the last place you stored fat is the first area to go; while the first place you stored it will be the last to go.

How many times have we all lost weight everywhere, except for that one annoying spot? That hated area is usually the lower abs for men and the hips/thighs for women. But know that if you stick to my program, even the troubled areas will get better. It's just a matter of time and hard work *on your entire body*.

You need to get the notion out of your head that you can spot-reduce. Consider that you only burn nine calories for every 20 crunches performed. So if you're 30 pounds overweight, how is just doing crunches going to give you better abs? You'd have to do 2,000 crunches to burn 900 calories, and a pound of fat contains 3,500 calories. Do you get it now?

You need to follow a *complete* exercise and nutrition program if you want to achieve a better midriff.

CHAPTER 2

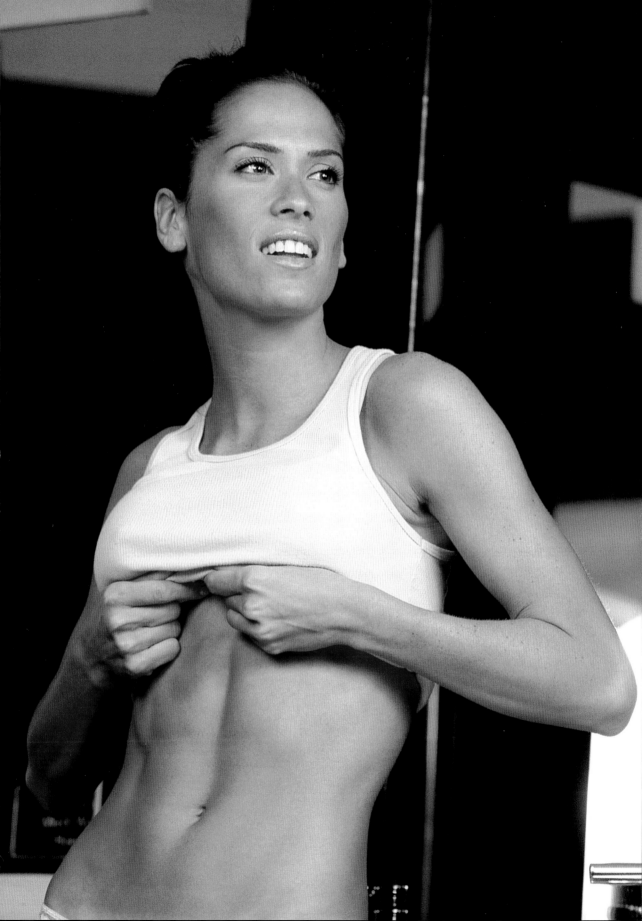

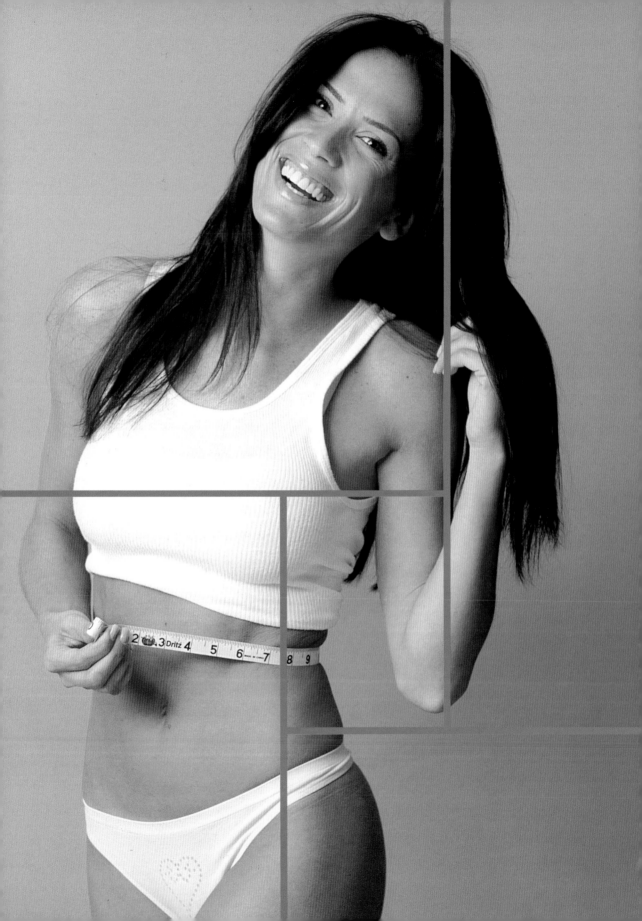

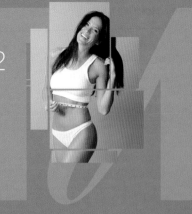

MISCONCEPTIONS ABOUT ABS

The biggest cause of mind-boggling frustration when it comes to obtaining the perfect stomach is misinformation and unrealistic expectations—and this could very well be what's keeping you from achieving your goals.

Although there are numerous books on the market that detail the right program to follow, people still cling to old-fashioned and improper techniques to get the desired six-pack. So in this chapter, we'll sort through all those myths surrounding your abs and set you free from them once and for all.

Myth: "Ab exercises will remove fat in my midsection."

Fact: This one is my favorite. We already talked about how spot-reducing doesn't work in the previous chapter, but allow me to remind you: The body dumps excess weight systematically and holistically, not one body part at a time. Remember that you need to remove excess fat on your stomach in order to see defined abs—and the only way you're going to do this is by following a low-calorie diet and beginning a weight-resistance program while adding cardio-vascular exercise.

You can choose to just do thousands of sit-ups a day . . . the end result will be that you'll get sore. Sure, you'll probably develop muscles, but they'll still be under your fat. This is our mantra: *Spot-reducing doesn't work.* Say it over and over again until you believe it. Remember that 2,000 crunches burns 900 calories, and you'll probably need to call an ambulance; however, if you do 30 minutes of cardio (depending on your intensity), you can easily burn 300 to 500 calories. Now that's a smart deal.

Myth: "I can eat doughnuts, pizza, or whatever I want—as long as I do my abdominal exercises, I'll never get fat."

Fact: I can't write now because I'm laughing so hard! Sadly, millions of folks believe this. I love when I see people go from my neighborhood gym to the deli across the street. They work out hard . . . and then go grab muffins, cakes, potato chips, cheese, and other junk foods. Because they burned some calories at the gym, they think it's okay. Remember that what makes us fat is the total amount of calories we eat in a day. So if the number of calories we ingest is greater than what we're burning, then those extra calories will make themselves known in the form of fat. It doesn't matter how many crunches we do—the extra calories we didn't burn will start showing up on the scale.

Myth: "My trainer told me that I shouldn't do any weight training or ab exercises until I get down to my ideal body weight."

Fact: Your trainer needs a wake-up call. I strongly suggest following a weight-resistance regimen that includes ab exercises. You can't only diet and expect to have the body of your dreams—it just won't happen. Working out each body part will increase your muscle mass, which will raise your metabolic rate, ultimately helping the fat-burning process. The bottom line is that as you melt off those pounds, you want to look in the mirror and see a toned physique staring back at you. Reducing your calories but not working out your entire body won't make that happen.

I have no idea why you wouldn't want to train your stomach muscles during this process. You'll burn extra calories, and your abs will strengthen your new midsection. A strong core in the middle of your body will also reduce and prevent lower back pain, while making it easier to perform, and excel, at other exercises.

Myth: "Abs aren't the same as regular muscles."

Fact: This is a short reply, but an important one: Muscle is muscle, period. The abdominals should be trained the same as your legs, back, and chest—in other words, they shouldn't get special treatment.

Myth: "You have to train your abs every day if you want a six-pack."

Fact: Abdominal muscles can be overtrained just like any other body part. Anytime you exercise a muscle, its tissue breaks down; consequently, you need to give that muscle enough rest and recuperation in order to regenerate. If you refuse to listen to me and choose to train your abs every single day, let me tell you what will happen: Your overtraining will result in diminished gains, soreness, and minimal results. You also might get a nasty case of diarrhea that will put a damper on any extracurricular activities you plan on doing outside the gym.

Now for some good news: Your abs are being worked indirectly when you train other body parts. Go over to the triceps push-down bar and do a quick set—you'll also feel the burn in your abs as they get some side-training. So be smart and choose quality over quantity when you focus on this muscle group.

Myth: "If you want great abs, you have to do a lot of reps while training."

Fact: The abdominal muscles aren't physiologically different from any other muscle. Given that fact, let me pose this question: If you were training your chest, would you do three sets of 100 reps on the bench press? Abs should be approached in the same way, yet people feel as if they have to do huge amount of reps with this area. Part of the reason is that you might not be working it correctly or intensely enough. For example, if you have to do 50 reps of leg raises before you feel the burn, then you're doing something wrong. You need to slow down and not use your body's momentum to do the exercise correctly.

It's the same with abs. Be honest with yourself: Are you pulling your head forward on crunches? Are you using your body's momentum to complete your reps? Are you contracting your muscles as hard as you can on every set? The bottom line is that if you're training your abs correctly, then you'll feel an immediate burn. You won't have the energy or physical prowess to do high-rep sets. If it's too easy, check your form.

Myth: "If you want a great six-pack, then you have to train your abs for hours."

Fact: This is very similar to the high-rep myth. You'd never spend two hours training your back. In fact, you shouldn't train *any* body part for hours. If you're training your abs correctly, then you should be in and out of the gym in less than 20 minutes *maximum.*

More is not better when it comes to training. Your body needs proper rest, or you'll become overtrained and your workouts will be counterproductive. Short, intense sessions will put you on the road to faster gains. So tell that guy in the gym who's been on the same machine for two hours to get off. (Just kidding—don't pick fights at the gym.) Seriously, if you've watched an entire *Oprah* while doing your crunches, it's time to reevaluate your routine.

Myth: "Men and woman should train their abs differently."

Fact: That's complete hogwash. A woman has muscle, and a man has muscle, which is trained the same way—by using resistance. So, if a woman wants to build a lean, sexy midriff, then she's going to eat correctly, follow a cardiovascular program, and train her abs using the same exercise regimen a man would. God has done many beautiful things, but he hasn't created a separate crunch for a woman and a man.

So in this book, I've provided you with a unisex list. Woman shouldn't think that they're going to put on huge amounts of mass by doing the same exercises as their husbands or boyfriends. Men produce 50 to 100 times more testosterone than women, so the chances of gals achieving the same muscular gains as guys are impossible (unless someone's slipping steroids into your low-fat cereal).

Myth: "If I stop training my abdominal muscles, they'll turn to fat."

Fact: Muscles don't turn to fat—but they *will* atrophy when you don't train them. If you stay active and watch what you eat, you'll probably keep your abs even if you stop training because the less fat in the area, the sharper the muscles will look. Of course, if you stop working out, your abs probably won't look as sharp as they did when you did exercise. But if you stop exercising *and* start eating junk food, your new abs will disappear in a heartbeat. If you want to maintain or improve your midsection, the best way to do so is to follow your program in addition to a proper diet, and keep up with your cardio. Believe me, once you see the results, you won't want to stop.

Myth: "It will take me years to develop perfect abs. Why bother?"

Fact: No, it won't. As I mentioned in the last chapter, everyone has abdominals—you just have to find the right plan to reduce the fat so that you can see them. How fast you'll achieve this is based on a few things. The first component is how much fat is surrounding your ab area. If you're 200 pounds overweight, it will take longer to develop your abs, but it can be done. Obviously, if you have less body fat to lose, then your results will come faster.

Another important factor in developing abs is following the right plan, eating correctly, following a cardiovascular program, and adding weight training. If you just do one of these things, you'll have a harder time training your midsection. You need to stay on track and remain consistent—don't miss workouts or make up rules to skip exercises along the way. Please don't think that just because you did 30 minutes of cardio, it entitles you to a bag of M&M's. And don't discount genetics: Different body types develop at different rates. It might take you a little more time or effort than the next person. Don't worry—you'll still see results. You get out of it what you put into it.

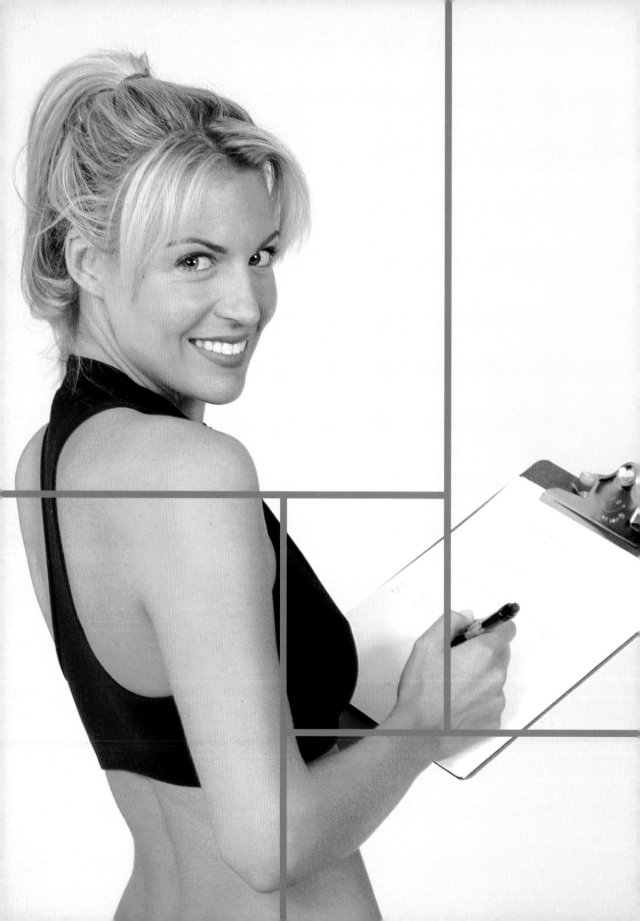

CHAPTER 3

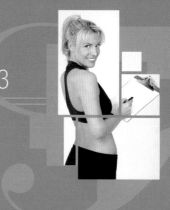

GOALS

Most people I meet say that they have fitness goals, but they're more like wishes or dreams. I want you to approach your workout in a much more practical way. For example, let's say that you're going to drive cross-country on vacation. You probably wouldn't just get in the car one morning and wing it—instead, you'd do some planning beforehand so that your intention of reaching your destination wouldn't just be a dream, but a reality. Well, it's the same thing with fitness. You need a plan so that you won't keep moving in an aimless fashion and never really get there.

First, you must realize why you want to achieve your goal. There are people out there who are happy size 20s, and they don't want to make any physical changes to their bodies. That's certainly their choice (although I do worry about their health). When individuals like this have come to me for advice in the past, I've told them that it's not always about having the six-pack—it's about creating a version of themselves that maximizes their optimal health and energy.

Yet some clients tell me that they're afraid to even think of making major changes. They'll say, "Frank, I just don't know how to begin. And what if I fail?" I tell them to forget about that, since each step they make toward a goal is a major success.

So what's the first step? I'd like you to decide why you want to follow a fitness program. Do you want to improve your athletic performance, enhance your current state of health, increase your energy levels, create a new and improved body, or better your self-esteem?

By setting goals and measuring your accomplishments, you'll quickly feel proud of yourself as you see what you can do. This will give you an incredible jolt of self-confidence that can extend to other areas in your life.

LET'S TAKE A MOMENT TO TALK ABOUT EXPECTATIONS. We've already picked apart the flood of advertisements out there that promote an unrealistic idea about what you can achieve. Don't be swayed into thinking that you have to match the accomplishments of those "before and after" ads.

It's also a good idea not to focus on how your best friend looks six months after losing 50 pounds, and forget about those movie stars who claim that they don't work out at all but just naturally have amazing figures. Who cares? Just worry about achieving your personal best. You only have to fulfill your own expectations.

Likewise, you have to distinguish between what's feasible and what isn't when you're making a goal; otherwise, you're setting yourself up for major disappointment. In other words, if you're 100 pounds overweight and your goal is to have a six-pack in six weeks, that's not a very practical aim. However, if you want to lose 20 pounds in eight weeks, that could probably happen if you work really hard. Keep in mind that any goal you set has to be attainable in order for it to come to fruition. So, if you can't leap a building in a single bound or melt steel with your eyes, then you better realize—quickly—that you're human, and anything worthwhile takes time to accomplish when it comes to the human body.

Short-Term Goals

The best thing to do is to set a short-term goal and then reach it. In other words, don't think that you can lose 50 pounds in four weeks when you haven't trained in ten years. It also works the other way: Don't set a short-term goal that's too easy to accomplish, such as losing four pounds in a month or dropping your waist size from a 38 to a 37 in five weeks. Set a reasonable aim that you can accomplish safely in a realistic time frame. It's about walking before you run. Short-term goals also require immediate attention and force you to take action, while long-term objectives are often too far into the future, so there's no pressure to get started.

Let's say that your long-term goal is to have a six-pack. Even though you're currently 50 pounds overweight with a stomach as squishy as a jelly doughnut, you've decided that you're going to get those fabulous abs no matter what. Well, if we work on a short-term goal first and change it every 30 days, then each time you accomplish it, you'll be closer to your long-term goal. You'll also be looking and feeling better every time you need to set a new target.

Short-term goals also give you time to stop and evaluate your progress: If you're not losing enough weight or seeing the significant changes you wanted, then you can make the necessary adjustments to your program. This is a much better idea than waiting six months and realizing that you still haven't really started working toward your long-term aim.

This reminds me of my client Jimmy, a nice guy who had just graduated from college. During those four years, he'd packed on a few extra pounds from fast food and an overconsumption of beer . . . which he didn't notice until his new girlfriend pointed it out (much to his dismay) at a beach party. At that point, Jimmy began to obsess about losing his gut and making his girlfriend proud of him. He came to me weighing 200 pounds with 20 percent body fat. That percentage isn't so good for a man, so I wanted Jimmy to get down to 10 percent body fat in order to see his abs again.

"Jimmy, we need to set some short-term goals in order to accomplish the bigger ones," I told him.

"Well, my first goal is to lose 10 pounds," Jimmy said. "I also want to have more muscle tone in 30 days."

This sounded reasonable to both of us, so we got to work. Every Monday for a month, I'd evaluate Jimmy's progress by testing his body fat, weighing him, and taking his measurements. I'd also look closely at him to see if any physical changes were apparent—if he'd slacked off, I'd give him my best "let's get motivated" speech.

I'm happy to report that five months later, Jimmy's abs had never looked better, and he'd surpassed his wildest expectations. (He also found a new girlfriend who didn't pick on his body.) I credit his success to that first short-term goal of losing 10 pounds, which forced him to get started. His successes just paved the way for the big win.

OF COURSE, IT'S VERY EASY to fall off the wagon. We lead incredibly stressful lives trying to balance work and family, so it's no wonder that fitness goals are easily shoved to the side. Some of us even lose track of them altogether. We're only human, right? If you feel as if your goal is slipping away, then it's time to step back, take a deep breath, and refocus.

The first thing to do is remind yourself why you set the goal in the first place. There was a reason why you wanted to lose weight and achieve that six-pack—are those reasons gone now? I'll bet that you just buried them because you got busy.

It's time to start again and dig up your goal. Recommit yourself, and envision what you'll look like when you reach it. Think of how good you'll feel—imagine what it will be like when you're a healthier person. I'm figuring that would make anyone feel pretty happy.

When your commitment starts to fade, you need to refocus and get back on track. A setback is only temporary, and achieving your long-term goal is just a matter of successfully completing a series of short-term goals along the way. So, you won't make any progress just sitting around thinking about starting a workout program a week from now—you need to take action today.

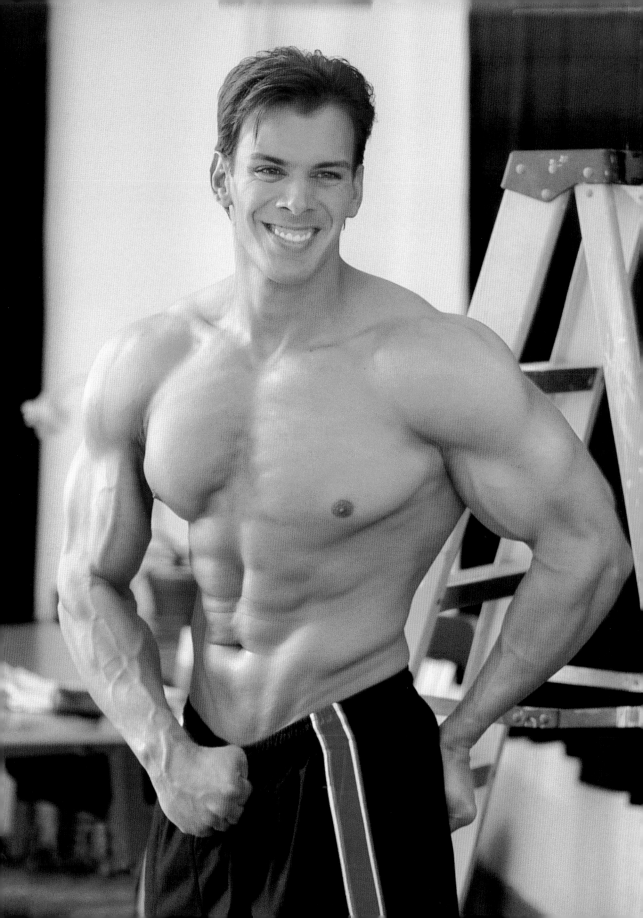

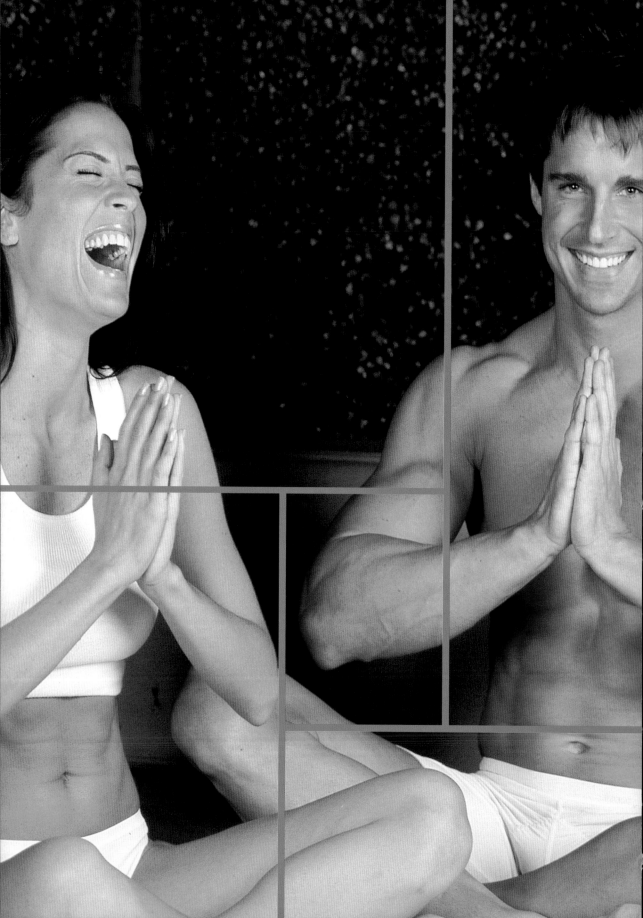

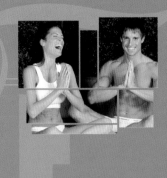

THE MIND-BODY CONNECTION

I'm no psychiatrist, and even though I've seen every episode of the TV show *Frasier,* I'm still not qualified to tell you how you should live your life. However, I *can* tell you how to get the most out of your training sessions. All you have to do is use your most important tool: your mind.

A gym owner once told me that every January he has about 2,000 people enroll because they swear that *this* is the year they'll finally get in shape . . . but come March, about a thousand of them are never to be seen again. These individuals quit for a variety of reasons, including no parking at the gym, dirty bathrooms, or an ex-girlfriend or boyfriend who works out there, too.

Of course, the most common reason that people go AWOL is that they're not mentally ready to accept a change in their lives.

Getting in shape means modifying the way you eat, trying new foods, eating at different times, avoiding fast-food restaurants, going to a gym, incorporating weight training, figuring out a cardio routine, and committing to a new way of life. It's a big deal, as is any lifestyle modification. There are folks who jump into these changes with both feet and the best intentions in the world, but I wonder if they're really prepared mentally to stay with their programs. That's what we'll tackle in this chapter.

Positive Visualization

If you plan on being successful when it comes to your fitness goals, then you need to remove any negative feelings or thoughts you have before you even begin. If you believe that you're going to fail, then it's inevitable that you will. You see, the information you relay to your subconscious has a huge impact on determining the results of anything you try.

Before you start any program, I strongly suggest that you make a positive change when it comes to your thought patterns. I want you to imagine how you'll feel with that washboard stomach you've been after for years. Now, start thinking about how your new abs will look: Visualize their separation, muscularity, and tautness. Once you have this image, you can use it to consciously create positive images in your head that will help you stay motivated and be an important tool in achieving your goals.

I teach this visualization technique to all my clients, and it works: Some people have a problem creating the images in their heads, so they use a photo of someone they want to emulate. That's fine, because the most important thing is creating a specific image for your abs. For example, my client Joan would stare at a photo of singer/actress Grace Jones from the movie *Conan the Destroyer* each time she didn't feel like going to the gym, and it really inspired her. Use whatever motivates *you* to reach your goals—it's your choice, and a very personal and individual thing.

Positive visualization must be practiced often in order for it to be effective. So let those inspirational images you've found repeatedly sink into your head until you start believing that you'll reach your goal. Use this method before and after you train to motivate you to go to the gym, and then plan to go back the next day. This doesn't have to become an obsession—just make sure that you're thinking about these images and how they inspire you to make positive changes.

Controlled Breathing

Here's one of the most common questions tossed my way: "When should I breathe during an exercise?"

My answer is an easy one: "Breathe in when exerting, and breathe out when you're done with a rep."

I remember seeing a man at my gym pass out during a set of squats. He was doing a 30-rep set and held his breath the whole time, until he finally collapsed. Fortunately, he wasn't hurt, but it was a good lesson. Obviously, you never want to prevent your brain and body from getting oxygen during exercise. If you do so, you'll faint—and in extreme cases, you could die.

Proper breathing is not only significant when training, but it can also be a great way to attain a relaxed state. If you've ever watched a boxer before he gets into the ring, you've probably noticed the coach telling him to take a few deep breaths to relax so that the fighter doesn't let his aggression race out of control. Or if you've ever been to an acting class, you know that the first thing the instructor teaches you is how to breathe properly, so you'll become more relaxed before your performance. (It's also a very helpful approach to stage fright.) In other words, it's all about "in with the good air, and out with the bad."

Let's try an experiment. Get in the most comfortable position you can. If that means standing or hanging upside down in a closet, that's fine—whatever works for you is perfect. Now, start to focus on your breathing for one to two minutes. (Take longer if you don't feel yourself relaxing.) Inhale on a count of five and exhale on the count of five. When you breathe in, I want you to think of the positive mental images we just discussed . . . think about that image, along with all the good things associated with it. When you breathe out, let go of any negative thoughts. Dismiss any reservations or fears, as well as anything that's going to impede you from achieving your goals. Just toss them aside with a breath.

I do this exercise for 20 minutes a day, but you can do it for as long as it takes for you to feel more relaxed and centered. I can't even begin to tell you how much better you'll feel when your mind is emptied of all its negativity. Make practicing your breathing a regular part of your day, for it will help you stay focused on your goals and is a great stress reliever.

Mantras (Power Phrases)

Now that you know how to do controlled breathing, you can add a little twist to your session with mantras. These are phrases that you create to help counteract any negative thoughts you might have. An example would be: "I am a winner." There's no doubt that this is a strong and powerful phrase. However, a phrase such as, "I think I can—tomorrow is a new day," is just not strong enough.

I want you to get into the habit of using these mantras when you feel doubts cropping up. Keep saying your phrase over and over when negative feelings arise—by doing so, you'll turn the doubt into self-confidence.

You can say your mantra anytime, but I've found that it works especially well during controlled-breathing exercises. I like to inhale, say my phrase in my head, and then exhale. This makes for an extremely positive breathing session, since I feel more motivated and free of self-doubt.

So, what's my mantra? "I am a success." It's simple, effective, and very positive—make sure that your mantra is the same.

Progressive Relaxation

If you want to take your relaxation to a whole new level, you should try a method called *progressive relaxation,* which is great for treating stress and anxiety. I have a friend who can get into a relaxed mental state no matter where he is or what's going on around him. The guy even fell asleep at a football game with 80,000 people around him screaming, "Jets!" Now that's a loose guy.

Basically, progressive relaxation is the active unwinding of each part of the body, one part at a time—while keeping your entire body in a relaxed state as you move on to each individual area. This practice works because of the relationship between your muscle stress and emotional stress. When you're in a state of emotional suffering, you routinely tense your muscles, so our goal here is to "de-tense." The steps are simple:

1. Find a quiet room. Turn off the TV and block out any outside noises.

2. Make sure that your body parts are comfortably supported (lie on the couch or bed, etc.).

3. Wear the most comfortable loose clothing you own—nothing that restricts you.

4. Do this for 15 minutes at the same hour every day, which is your time to master this technique.

5. Stay focused on all the sensations that come from letting go of tension, and be aware of your body.

6. Concentrate on relaxing all your muscles. You should be giving 100 percent attention to those muscles—doing so will make it very difficult to think about the everyday, stressful problems that cause you anxiety.

7. Once you're completely relaxed, start focusing on specific muscle groups. One at a time, start tensing and relaxing each group while breathing slowly and deeply. You should tighten each muscle group for 20 seconds at a time and start working from the top to the bottom of your body.

It takes a lot of practice to master this technique, but stick with it. You'll reach a heightened state of calmness that you've never achieved before.

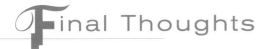

Final Thoughts

All the methods that I've discussed in this chapter will help you achieve a heightened mental state, as well as assisting you in reaching your goal of obtaining a flatter midsection faster.

Some people think that these visualization techniques are hokey because they don't believe in the mind-body connection. For all you nonbelievers out there, I wonder: Have you ever had to mentally prepare yourself for a big meeting? Have you ever had to give yourself a pep talk before a big sporting event? Have you ever had to psych yourself up before asking someone out? Well, why should achieving your goal of great abs be any different? You have to mentally prepare and continually keep your mind focused on your goal—which all the techniques in this chapter will help you do.

Never dismiss the mind-body connection, because the mind is a very powerful thing.

CHAPTER 5

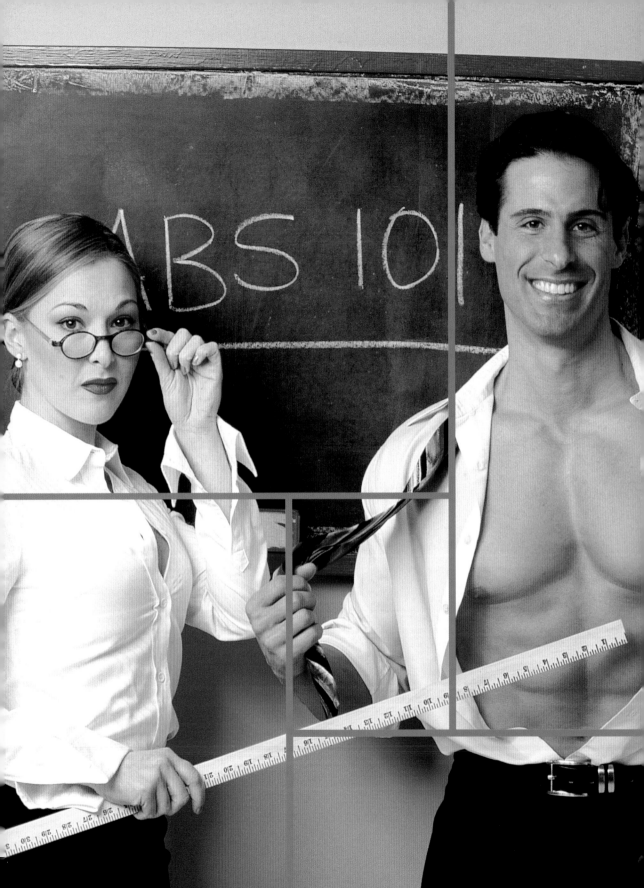

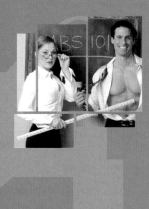

ABS 101

It's time to get a quick lesson in the anatomy of your abs before we start training them. You won't be a candidate for medical school by the end of his chapter, but you *will* know the basics—and this is helpful, because knowledge is power.

Whenever I try something new, I always learn as much about that particular subject as I can. If you're going to spend the rest of your life doing ab exercises, then you should know what you're working on so diligently. Knowing the basics will also help you visualize the muscle you'll be training, so you can become more in tune with your exercises. This will translate into your having a much more effective workout.

There are four muscle groups that make up the abdominal area; these groups allow the body to lower and raise the torso and twist from side to side. Let's get started with the first group, the rectus abdominis.

Rectus Abdominis

Rectus means "straight" and *abdominis* means "abdominal": this is the large muscle in front of your abdomen that helps in the regular breathing movement and sustains the muscles of the spine when lifting. It also keeps abdominal organs such as the intestines in place.

The rectus abdominis runs from your sternum to your pubic bone—if you're genetically gifted, then you'll have six segments (or boxes) of muscle above your belly button and a pancake-flat sheath below it. Don't worry if you only have two or four boxes, and don't be alarmed if your boxes aren't exactly aligned—this is all based on your genetics, so you can't create another box. Likewise, there's nothing you can do if one box is higher than another.

People don't realize that the rectus abdominis is one muscle; in other words, when you hear discussions about your lower and upper abs, that isn't really correct. However, it is true that different ab exercises will cause more of a sensation in a certain area than others. For example, if you were to do a standard crunch, then you'd feel it in your middle- to upper-ab region; but if you were to do a lying leg raise, then you'd feel more of a burn in the lower part of your abdomen.

External and Internal Obliques

The obliques are more commonly known as "love handles," and most people don't know that they're actually muscles. Now, that doesn't mean that if you have a huge set of obliques you're really pumped—more than likely, it means that you're carrying excess fat.

The obliques are very important for balancing out your entire midsection. After all, how many people have you seen with a great six-pack that have fat obliques? I'd say not one. Cosmetically, the obliques are important in framing out your entire midsection; while, functionally, they play a big role in sports. Anytime you twist your trunk, whether you're hitting a baseball, shooting a puck, or swinging a golf club, your obliques come into play, so you need to make sure that they're trained effectively. *Do not neglect these muscles.*

Your abdominals are supported by your external and internal obliques. The external obliques are the more prominent of the two, and they're the largest of the abdominal muscles. They're found lateral to the rectus abdominis, meaning to your side. They originate from the external surfaces of the lower eight ribs, and insert into the anterior half of the outer lip of the *iliac crest* and the *aponeurosis abdominal wall.* The function of the external oblique is to aid in the twisting or turning of the trunk. This means that if you twist your trunk to the right, then your left external oblique is stimulated; if you twist left, your right external oblique is stimulated.

The internal obliques originate from the *lumbar spine fascia, anterior iliac crest,* and the lateral two thirds of the *inguinal ligament,* and they insert into the 9th through 12th ribs and the *linea alba.* The internal oblique helps aid the trunk in twisting or turning in the same direction.

Transverse Abdominis

The transverse muscle holds your gut firm and flat. It's a slim sheet of muscle running along the sides of the abs, which fuses connective tissue behind it. The fibers run across the stomach, join into the rear area of the abs, and wrap around the sides of the body. They attach along the rib cage and into the back muscles.

As the *transverse abdominis* contracts, it compresses the internal organs. This helps the lungs to exhale, and lets the body perform the normal process of elimination. Basically, these are the muscles that allow you to suck in your stomach. So the next time you're at the beach and a good-looking guy or girl passes by, thank your transverse abdominis as you hold in your gut.

Less cosmetically speaking, these muscles also play an important role in stabilizing the lower back and keeping good posture. So, if you train these muscles, you're more likely to have a flatter stomach, better posture, and a more stable pelvis and lower back.

Spinal Erectors (Lower Back)

Unless you're totally in tune with your body, the last time you saw this muscle was in the dressing-room mirror at the department store. So now I'd like you to take your hand and place it on your lower back, just above your butt. These are your spinal erectors, or the muscles that straighten your body when you bend forward and lend a hand in allowing your body to twist.

I'm going to leave out the rest of the medical jargon—you get the idea. Nevertheless, you might be asking yourself why I'm talking about the back in a book on abs. Well, training this area has many benefits, including improving your posture and strengthening your core.

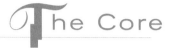 # The Core

Isn't it funny how all of a sudden certain words break into the fitness world? We've already added *ripped, six-pack, spotter,* and *crunch* to our current vocabulary. Well, the new word today is *core.*

Core strength refers to the muscles in your abs and back and their ability to support your spine and keep your body stable and balanced. All of our movements are powered by our torsos, so it's important to work the core—that's all it means.

I know it gets confusing when people start taking out exercise balls and start ranting and raving about doing core-specific exercises. There's no need to be confused: Working on this area simply means strengthening your abs and back in order to support your body during weight-resistance exercises. In order to strengthen your core, you'll need to target certain muscle groups in your workout.

Later in this book, you'll receive all the ab and back exercises you need to achieve the strongest core possible and create a better overall physique. But now, in Part II, we're going to take the time to work on three principles that will ensure that you see results: nutrition, cardio, and other fat burners.

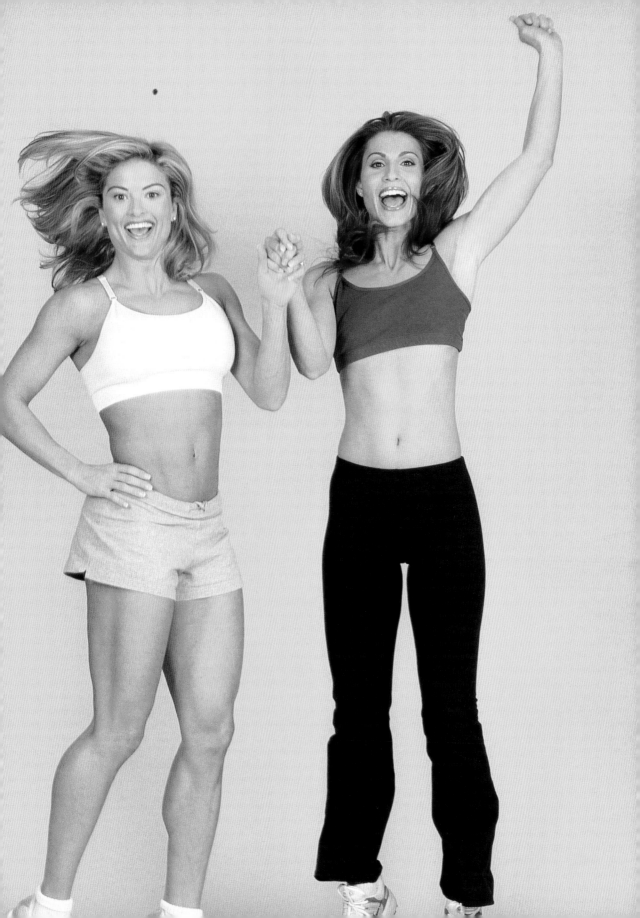

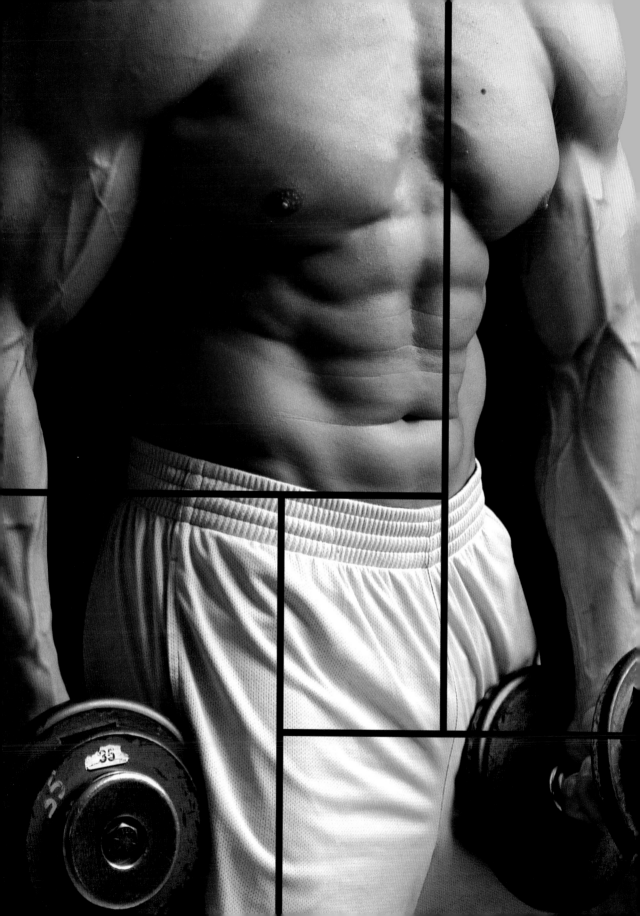

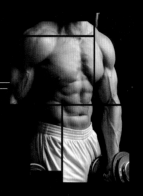

PART II

The Three Principles to Building Abs

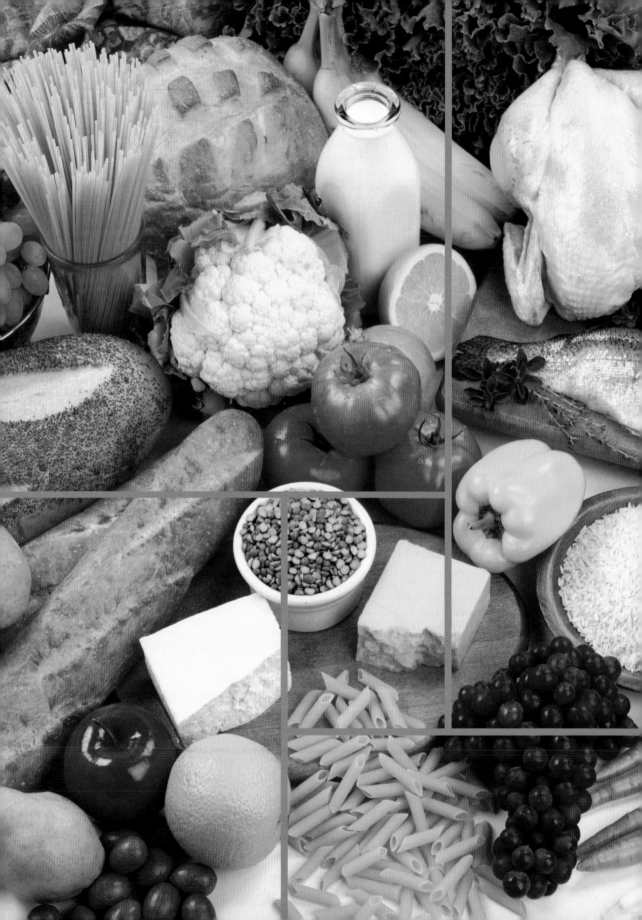

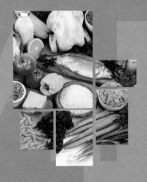

NUTRITION

Unfortunately, unless your body-fat percentage is low, then the only six-pack you're going to see is at the grocery store. That is, you can't just eat what you want and still hope to have a flat midsection. I'm sorry, but you're going to have to put down those fast-food burgers, throw away those bakery delights, shun your local ice-cream vendor, and keep reading this book.

What can I say about diets? For the past 15 years, I've been involved in the fitness industry, and during that time, I'll bet that a thousand diets have come onto the scene. Most of those plans only offer false hope and fuel unrealistic expectations in the minds of their followers. Well, I've got news for you: Eating correctly isn't about following the latest trend for a few weeks until you lose five pounds—it's about embracing fitness and living healthy as a lifestyle. It's a full-time, long-term commitment, and you can't treat your eating plan like a short-term inconvenience.

Remember that it doesn't matter how many hours you spend in the gym if you're not eating right, since you'll never achieve optimal results. Your entire program's success is contingent on how well you do in the eating department, and there are two things you need to know first: basic nutrition and how to make smart food choices.

In this chapter, I'll give you a brief and simple lesson on eating correctly. I'm not going to try to dazzle you with scientific terminology, nor will I give you useless stats about food and its chemical makeup—you can find all that on the Internet or in your local library. What I want to share with you is information you can actually understand and use. So, in this section, you'll learn everything you need to know about nutrition to use in conjunction with the rest of the plan in order to achieve the midsection of your dreams. This is definitely not a chapter you want to skip.

As I like to say: "Get your learn on."

Body Fat

It's pretty funny to me that when people talk about obtaining a flat stomach or a six-pack, the words *body fat* rarely come into the conversation. Instead, I'm more likely to hear, "I need to lose 20 pounds to get back in my bikini," or "If I lost 15 pounds, I'd get rid of these love handles." Well, I've got a big reality check for those of you who don't understand the importance of losing body fat instead of pounds.

Let's say you weigh 150 pounds and your body fat is 20 percent. You decide that you want to lose ten pounds for the summer, so you're going to drastically cut your calories while reducing your carbs down to zero. You do just that for two weeks—however, even though the scale indicates that you've lost ten pounds, your stomach doesn't look any tighter and your body doesn't appear more toned. You decide to get a skin-caliper test, only to discover that your body fat is exactly the same at 20 percent. Why didn't it go down, too?

It's important that you understand the following: If you choose to cut out carbs completely or reduce your calories too much, then your body is going to lose a combination of fat, water, and muscle. When you get on the scale and you weigh ten pounds less, that's not going to be ten pounds of *just* fat. This is a very common scenario, since most people still believe that the best way to lose weight is to stop eating.

In reality, the best way to lose weight is to follow a balanced diet that consists of protein, carbs, and fat. And just losing weight won't translate into a ripped six-pack—anyone with a flat torso will tell you that the key is *lowering your body fat*. In other words, unless your body fat is around 10 percent for men and 15 percent for women, you won't have visible abs. So my advice to anyone seeking that dream midsection is to buy some skin calipers and test your body fat once a week. Use the mirror to evaluate your progress—stop living and dieting by what the scale reads.

Diet Plans

Not long ago, I was in the gym listening to a woman talk about her new liquid diet. She was drinking this gross concoction for 72 hours to lose weight. I begged her to stop. Yes, she might lose a few pounds, but the diet is so vitamin-and-mineral deficient that it could only lead to temporary weight loss. As soon as this woman starts eating regular foods, she'll gain the weight back. And she's certainly not going to just drink her disgusting juice forever.

It's not your fault if you've been suckered into trying one of these useless diets. There are so many out there now that it's difficult to find the right one. It's almost to the point that if you're not on a trendy eating plan then something must be wrong with you. In fact, I was at a local restaurant the other day and a friend ordered a sandwich on whole-wheat bread. You should have seen the reaction of the other people! It was as if the guy had just spit on the table because he was eating bread. Come on, now—carbs aren't going to be the death of us (even though there are many people who treat them as if they're poisonous).

Meanwhile, if you took the average body-fat percentage of the folks judging this man because of his sandwich, it would definitely have been in excess of 20 percent. They weren't exactly fit people; and you should have seen what they were eating—bacon, cheese, and pork—now *that's* an unhealthy diet. If any lives needed saving, it would have been one of these individuals.

Misinformation, lack of common sense, and an insane diet plan all contribute to people failing to lose their excess weight. Again, trendy diets might make you drop a few pounds at first, but they rarely give you enough energy to perform your cardio, weight training, and ab exercises. I could come up with the Frank Sepe M&M's Diet: All you eat is three bags of M&M's every single day. Sure, you'll lose a few pounds, but it will mostly be water weight. You won't gain any new muscle, and your abs will remain flabby. (Your teeth will probably also rot!)

My advice is to forget the trendy diets. Which ones have ever changed your life in the past? I know that it's convenient to look for a quick and easy solution, but the only answer is to eat right and work out *throughout your entire life.* I don't recommend zero carbs or diets that focus on one food group—but I do advocate hard work and common sense.

You need to follow an eating program that includes protein, carbohydrates, and fat if you plan on changing your body for the better over the long run. Think of it like breaking a plate into three equal sections (and please make sure that it isn't the size of a pizza pan—the general rule of thumb is an eight-inch plate for men and a six-inch plate for women). In one section of the plate, you'll have a protein source such as chicken, salmon, or turkey. The second section will have an equal amount of complex carbohydrates such as potatoes, grains, and the like. And section three will contain a green veggie such as broccoli, asparagus, and so on. Now *that's* a balanced meal. When I sit down to eat, whether I'm at home or in a restaurant, that's my basic meal plan.

A well-balanced eating program is crucial to your success. When you eat like this, you increase your level of health; achieve your goals in a safe, healthy, and sensible way; enjoy food; and keep your energy and mental state in a positive zone. It boils down to embracing fitness as a lifestyle and not a short-term experience—you must keep this in mind as you pursue physical success.

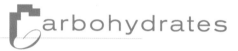arbohydrates

When did *carb* become such a four-letter word? Not since the movie *Gigli* has anything gotten such a bad rap. Everyone should just slow down for a second, take a deep breath, and stop carb bashing. Oh, and have a sweet potato while you're at it!

Carbohydrates are essentially either sugars or starches, and they're made up of three elements: carbon, hydrogen, and oxygen. Carbs break down into glucose molecules (bear with me here), and when you exert yourself physically, carbs become fuel for your muscles and brain functions. They also supply energy for bodily functions including breathing and the pumping of your heart.

Who needs carbs? How about the human race! Carbohydrates provide the most easily accessible energy source for your body. Imagine what would happen if you didn't eat carbs and headed off to the bedroom for a little loving. You'd lack the necessary energy to go that extra mile. Let me put it another way: Without enough carbs in your diet, your body will use an alternate, less efficient path that won't give you the same energy and will instead leave you tired and weak. When it comes to brain function, breathing, and energy . . . well, those are areas I don't want to be weak in.

Now here's the bad news: If your body has more glucose (how your body converts carbs) than it can use as energy, the excess is converted to fat. If you eat too many carbohydrates and don't burn them off during exercise or your daily life, you're going to gain weight.

Carbs are not your enemy—eating *too many* and *the wrong kind* is what gets you into trouble. In other words, if your daily menu consists of cake, cookies, muffins, potato chips, candy, white bread, and ice cream, and the only form of exercise you get is walking to the fridge, then you're going to become fat.

Carbohydrates are broken down into two forms: *simple* and *complex.* Simple carbohydrates contain table sugar *(sucrose)* or natural sugar *(fructose,* found in fruit; and *lactose,* found in milk), corn syrup, and a variety of concentrated sweeteners. Your dentist loves simple sugars because they've bought him his Mercedes.

When you eat too many simple sugars, your body produces insulin to counteract the effect. This results in a fast drop in your blood-sugar level, which will leave you feeling lethargic. Unfortunately, that simple boost you get from the sugar will be short-lived. (This is why athletes chug Gatorade during sporting events—for that quick burst of energy.)

Complex carbs, on the other hand, are released slowly into the bloodstream, thereby providing your body with a long-burning fuel supply. They also won't cause the sudden outpouring of insulin that simple carbs do. There's no sudden crash, and your body won't have huge cravings for food (which you'll suffer when you eat simple carbohydrates). The reason you don't get these side effects with complex carbs is because there's a low-energy release, the body's blood-sugar level remains stable, and you avoid the excessive high and low blood-sugar levels brought on by simple carbs.

As an athlete/bodybuilder, I've found that the best sources of complex carbohydrates are potatoes, whole grains, and green vegetables. Complex carbs are also filled with an abundance of vitamins, minerals, and fiber, so when compared to simple carbs, they're definitely the more nutritious of the two.

Here's a quick refresher:

1. Simple carbohydrates include foods that contain the most basic form of carbs: sugar (also known as sucrose, fructose, and lactose). These include white sugar, brown sugar, confectioner's sugar, corn syrup, honey, maple syrup, and molasses. So, basically any food that tastes good—such as candy, cookies, doughnuts, milk, and yogurt—are considered simple carbs because they're filled with sugar.

2. Complex carbohydrates typically contain more fiber, and have a more complex chemical structure that takes longer to digest. *Starch* is the common term for complex carbs, which include breads, cereals, crackers, rice, pasta, potatoes, corn, peas, lima beans, and legumes (such as chickpeas, garbanzo beans, kidney beans, and lentils).

Which Is Better: Complex or Simple?

If you're trying to get in shape and create a healthier body, then you should consume more complex carbs. I'm not saying that all simple carbs are bad, but I *am* saying that you need fewer of them than you do the complex. Too many simple carbs will result in raising your cholesterol; increasing your fat percentage; and possibly, over time, contributing to adult-onset (type 2) diabetes. So, if you're going to ingest a simple sugar, then do it in the form of something natural like milk—that is, don't just grab a doughnut.

Of course, complex carbs will also make you fat if you eat too many of them, but at least they contain more minerals, vitamins, and fiber than simple carbs. Complex carbs are necessary for your overall health—they're an essential macronutrient for people who exercise, as well as for sedentary people. All carbs trigger the release of insulin, a hormone needed to help amino acids enter muscle cells. If you exercise and decide not to eat carbs, you won't be able to train very hard, your energy levels will be low (despite how much fat you eat), and your body will have a difficult time recovering properly from your exercise regimen.

The key to eating carbohydrates is to use them up. If you're going to exercise, then the best time to eat carbs is before you exercise—but make sure they're complex, as they'll provide energy and build up your glycogen stores, which will become depleted during your workout. However, you will need a small amount of simple carbs immediately after your workout in order to start the recovery process.

Remember: Carbs are not the enemy. The reason people get fat from them is overindulgence and inactivity.

Sugar Is Kryptonite to Abs

If you ever want to see your abs, then you need to stay away from sugary snacks and drinks. Besides containing sugar, those tasty snacks contain a lot of useless calories. If you were to have one doughnut and one of those delicious Starbucks Frappuccinos, you've just added an extra 1,000 calories to your day. And if you do this every day, then that's 7,000 extra calories a week. That's a lot of calories to work off at the gym!

However, if you were to eat six egg whites and half a cup of oatmeal, that would add up to around 300 calories—which would consist of protein, carbs, and good fat. Now, you might say, "I can't eat six eggs. That's insane!" Yet you might find that you can pack away 1,000 calories of sugar at one sitting. Of course sugar tastes better, but it wreaks havoc on your insulin levels and promotes fat storage. All those Twinkies, cupcakes, and doughnuts you eat show up in the form of fat. They find a nice home around your waist or hips, or in another spot where you're genetically predisposed to gaining fat. Next time you look in the mirror and see a roll of fat, you can thank all your prepackaged and sugary sweet treats for welcoming that addition to your waistline.

That reminds me of this client I had, who used to have a glass of apple-cranberry juice for breakfast every day. After all, she told me, it was only 200 calories, and she couldn't eat a solid meal in the morning.

I said that the calories weren't the problem—the problem was that her drink contained 34 grams of sugar. So I asked her, "Why don't you just have a protein shake?"

"Oh, I don't want to gain weight," she replied.

This woman was operating from misinformation. Her drink contained fructose (otherwise known as sugar), and that set up a perfect environment for fat storage. The bottom line is that if you eat sugar, you're going to get fat and never see your abs. Be smart and make the right choices, and you'll have the sweetest midriff you can imagine.

Protein

If you don't eat protein, then you won't retain or build any lean mass. For all of you who believe that protein is going to make you fat, you're sadly mistaken. Protein is the only nutrient that actually feeds the lean muscle tissue in your body—so if you don't make it part of your daily eating program, then you'll never have that toned, flat midsection you're wishing for. Remember that the abdominals need protein just like any other muscle.

I can't forget a client of mine who refused to eat protein; instead, he lived on pasta and fruit. He trained six days a week and didn't miss a session for eight weeks. Nevertheless, he ended up looking like a scaled-down version of when he started. He lost muscle, but he wasn't toned—he just weighed less. Now, if he'd eaten protein during those eight weeks, he would have enhanced his muscle tone.

The next time you're at the supermarket, I want you to remember what I've said here and purchase some protein-rich foods, including chicken, turkey, or egg whites. (You can also pick up some protein powder—I use those made by MET-Rx or Worldwide.) You need protein to build a stronger, healthier, and leaner body.

Fats

There are certain fats that you want to stay away from, including those that are saturated, hydrogenated, and oxidized (this includes trans-fatty acids, too). These tend to be found in butter, French fries, doughnuts, candy, and so forth, and they're the ones that cause you to gain weight. You're much better off without them.

However, not all fats are created equal. Monosaturated and omega-3 fats found in foods such as peanut butter; nuts and seeds; flaxseed, canola, and olive oils; and fish such as salmon have many benefits, including reducing the risk of cardiovascular disease and providing essential fatty acids and fat-soluble vitamins that are required for good health. So if you're deficient in essential fatty acids, then you'll be interfering with the function of every cell in your body—in fact, the cell membrane is comprised mostly of essential fats. Who knew that fat was so good for you?

Fat can also be used as an additional energy source, as well as being crucial to the maintenance and condition of your hair, skin, and nails, as well as your energy levels. Of course, this doesn't mean that you should wolf down a whole jar of Skippy—it just means that *in moderation,* fat is an essential and helpful nutrient.

By now you should have a basic idea of the nature of good nutrition, so it's time to move on to making smart food choices.

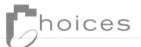
Choices

Whenever I'm asked what separates a person who has an incredible midsection from someone whose midriff resembles a vat of pizza dough, I say that the choices of when, what, and how much to eat is what makes the difference. In other words, if you pull into that drive-through in the middle of the night and feast on greasy fries and burgers, then you have to accept the fact that you're choosing to be out of shape. No one's putting a gun to your head and making you eat that slop—you're making the choice. You have to understand that what you choose to eat either has a positive or negative effect on your body; so if you eat poorly, then you'll never get those washboard abs, even if you train like a maniac.

It's like having a brand-new Ferrari and then putting tainted gas in it: It might still drive, but unless you fuel it with the right stuff, you won't get optimal performance out of the car. Similarly, it's time to put your bad eating habits behind you and start fresh. Just reading this chapter means that you're off to a good start, but I'm going to make it even easier for you because what follows are my best tips on how to make good food choices . . . which can then lead to a set of ripped abs.

TOP FOODS TO AVOID FOR A FLATTER STOMACH

- Soda (including diet sodas)—all that carbonation will just cause bloating
- Potato chips and packaged snack foods
- Processed baked goods, cakes, cookies, candy, and doughnuts
- Deep-fried foods
- Alcohol (it's extremely calorie-dense)
- Margarine and spreads
- Soups (they're high in sodium)
- Ice cream and cheese

TOP PROTEIN FOODS (IN NO PARTICULAR ORDER)

- Turkey
- Chicken
- Egg whites
- Beef (flank steak)
- Salmon
- Whitefish (halibut, cod, etc.)
- Swordfish
- Fat-free cottage cheese
- Beans and legumes
- Protein powder, such as MET-Rx

TOP CARBOHYDRATES (IN NO PARTICULAR ORDER)

- Vegetables (green leaf)
- Potatoes (baked or boiled)
- Sweet potatoes/yams
- Rice, brown or white
- Oatmeal or oats
- Grains (whole-grain pasta, etc.)

TOP FATS (IN NO PARTICULAR ORDER)

- Almonds
- Cashews
- Peanut butter
- Olive, corn, peanut, sesame, and canola oils
- Fish oil

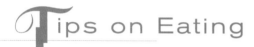ips on Eating

Tell me if this scenario sounds familiar: You catch your reflection in the mirror one day and notice that when you turn to the side, your stomach is sticking out a little farther than you'd like. That's when you remember this fantastic new diet book you heard about. You get in your car, drive down to the local bookstore, and purchase the plan—but before you get home, you stop and pick up an ice-cream cone or a muffin. Why not, right? You're starting your diet tomorrow. (Hey, we've all done it.) You get home, read your new book, and think, *This time I'm really going to do it.*

The next day, you hit the supermarket and pick up all the healthy foods you need. You might even buy a notebook to serve as a food journal. And you start your diet. You stay super strict on this eating program for a couple of weeks and start to look better. But for some reason, your stomach still looks distended. You blame genetics, but then you stumble upon a photo of yourself from a year ago, when your tummy was perfectly flat. It's time to get depressed . . . so you quit your useless diet and go on an eating binge that would make any sumo wrestler feel full. Does this sound familiar?

What you don't know is that certain foods and beverages on your new diet could be the reason that your stomach isn't looking its best. There's a tip list that follows that you can use to combat stomach bloat. You don't have to do everything on the list, but do try to avoid a few of these pitfalls. Remember that your genetic makeup is different from the next person's, so what's causing you to retain that water might be very different from what your neighbor's going through.

(It's also a good idea to discuss your dietary problems with your doctor before you make any changes to your eating habits. And try to find one who's in reasonably good shape—after all, you don't want nutritional advice from an overweight physician. Someone who doesn't practice what he preaches makes me say, "Hmm.")

Areas to Watch in Order to Reduce Stomach Bloating and Distention

1. Sugar-free foods. Do you know what *sugar free* means to me? It means that I better plan on being alone for the day or in a wide-open space outdoors. Most people pass gas after eating these foods, which are loaded with chemicals. The main ingredient in a lot of these sugar-free items is sorbitol, which doesn't digest well—at least not by me or most people I know. It produces gas, which in turn, causes bloating. If you're experiencing stomach bloating and you're eating sugar-free foods, this could be why. (By the way, the fact that a food is sugar free doesn't mean that it's *calorie* free. All calories add up, including those of the sugar-free variety.)

2. Alcohol. Let's try this scenario: You diet from Monday to Friday at 9 P.M., when you go out to your local bar with your friends to have a few cocktails. You worked hard all week, so you deserve this, right? I'm sure you do, but your abs don't deserve all that alcohol.

Keep in mind that just because it's a drink doesn't mean that it's calorie free. Some alcoholic drinks such as daiquiris can contain upwards of 500 calories! However, I'm not advising you to have a shot of vodka as a substitute: All booze—beer, wine, and spirits—has more than seven calories per gram, which means that it's extremely calorie-dense. And those excess calories have a funny way of showing up around your midsection.

Alcohol is also a natural diuretic, so it can have a dehydrating effect on your body, causing your stomach to bloat. There are people who can get away with having a few drinks a week, but I suggest that you strictly limit your booze intake if you want great abs. I never saw a wino with a six-pack, and I have yet to see a book that explains how you can achieve a fabulous beer belly.

3. Beans, fruits, and vegetables. We spoke about the gas caused by sugar-free items; well, there are other foods that could also cause your stomach to fill up with gas, including fruits, vegetables, and different types of beans. Some of these foods can cause extreme bloating and then gas because they contain complex sugars called *oligosaccharides.* Your body has a very difficult time digesting these sugars, so it produces intestinal gas that can swell your stomach for up to 24 hours after eating that food. This doesn't occur in everyone, but if you're at your wit's end because you've ruled out everything else, this could be the reason. I suggest cutting back on these items and then carefully monitoring your stomach patterns. Fruits, vegetables, and beans are all great foods that have a positive effect on your body when eaten moderately and correctly.

4. Sodium. Foods that are high in sodium cause stomach bloat—there's no way around it. If you plan on going to your local sushi restaurant and using tons of soy sauce, then you'll probably be taking in about 3,000 to 6,000 milligrams of sodium. That's a lot for one person.

Sodium also causes *edema,* which is the swelling of the hands and feet; plus, it spikes your blood pressure. I suggest that you keep a careful watch on your sodium intake by closely reading food labels. There are many edibles that contain high traces of sodium, and they could bloat your abs for weeks. For example, I suggest that you stay away from packaged foods, cured meats, soups, French fries, and sauces, which are notorious for containing tons of sodium. Try to eat fresh, natural foods instead.

5. Water/carbonated beverages. If you were stranded on a desert island, what would be the first thing you'd need to survive? No, not Ginger or Mary Ann—the answer is water. It's sad that so many of us shun water when it's the most important thing we put in our bodies. The problem is that we have too many drink options. We often opt for diet soda instead of water, which we think is okay because of the word *diet.* Yes, it's better than drinking a high-sugar beverage, but it's still a carbonated drink, which causes that pesky stomach bloating. The carbon dioxide inside the floating bubbles in your soda creates gas, which slows down stomach emptying and creates a big belly.

What you need to do is drink water because it helps you flush out the toxins and sodium in your body. In addition, lack of water in your system is also a cause of a bloated stomach. Drink at least 8 eight-ounce glasses of water in a day to ensure proper hydration. (Another note: I've been noticing all those low-carb beers and drinks popping up these days. You don't need them—again, they're just sources of unnecessary calories.)

6. Eating late at night. You may have fallen into the bad habit of eating too much late at night, and this is one of the worst things you can do to your body. If you ingest a lot of calories and then remain inactive (asleep) for eight hours, that food is just sitting in your stomach. You may wake up with a temporarily distended stomach—sooner or later that water bloat will become permanent fat.

If you're eating at night, stop doing so immediately and watch the magic begin on your stomach. Start eating your heavier meals in the morning so that you can burn those calories off during your daily activities and your workout. Follow this guideline: Eat breakfast like a king, lunch like a queen, and dinner like a pauper.

7. Increasing your fiber. If you're not eating enough fiber, then you're probably not going to the bathroom regularly, which can also cause your stomach to bloat. And not eating enough roughage is one of the main reasons you're not getting that ripped six-pack. You just have to find the right balance of fiber and add it to your diet slowly and consistently—eating too much will cause bloating and gas, so spread your intake over the course of the day. If you eat a bunch of fiber in one meal, you'll definitely get a bloated stomach. Some doctors say that you must eat 25 grams daily; if you're going to eat that much, then you should drink plenty of water to keep that food moving through your system.

8. Stress. It seems as if stress is the main cause of everything these days: It causes high blood pressure and leads to anxiety attacks and multiple other unhealthy conditions. But believe it or not, stress also causes bloating in the stomach area because it sets off the hormone *cortil,* which turns up your appetite and deposits fat around the organs of your abdomen. This happens because this area has more receptors for cortisol than any other cells in the human body.

Don't be a stress victim—read Chapter 4 on relaxation techniques. You have to rid yourself of this tension because the happier you are, the better chance you have of lowering those hormone levels and flattening out your stomach.

Your Personal Eating Plan

Now it's time to put together an eating program that will supply you with protein, carbohydrates, and fat. You need a diet that doesn't restrict your calories too much because you don't want to lose muscle as you're losing fat. The American Medical Association recommends that you don't go below 10 calories per body pound; and I'm here to tell you that those 1,000-calorie diets are doing more harm than good.

Remember that everyone has a different genetic makeup and responds differently to different diets. What works for your best friend might not work for you, and vice versa. It's only through trial and error that you'll find your perfect eating program.

THE EATING PROGRAM I SUGGEST is the one I wrote about in my first book, *The TRUTH.* It's a high-protein, moderate-carb, low-fat plan, which has helped thousands of people—including me—achieve their fitness goals . . . including washboard abs.

It's also a very simple plan. Basically, you'll be consuming one gram of protein and carbs for each pound of your current body weight, while the amount of fat you'll be eating is based on your body weight x .22. (I've included the formulas below to show you just how easy it is to put your plan together.)

This program will assure you enough protein to build muscle, enough carbs to fuel your workout, and enough good fats to keep your body functioning properly. However, you may need to make an adjustment or two as you go along. For example, if you start to lose more than two pounds a week after the first few weeks, you can gradually increase your calories to ensure that you don't lose any hard-earned muscle. Also, if you're very carb sensitive, then an option may be to increase your protein to 1.5 grams per body pound and drop your carbs to .75 per pound. The only way you're going to figure out that you need to make an adjustment is by following the initial program. And know that following this eating plan will definitely improve your abs.

Breaking Down Your Meals

When you start putting your program together, you need to remember that the times of eating three square meals a day are long gone—that's not the way to lose weight. Instead, you need to eat a minimum of four times a day, preferably even more. Small meals throughout the day, usually every two to three hours, will keep your blood-sugar level more constant, deter hunger, and stop binge eating. Eating consistent meals also helps convince your body and mind that you're not starving. It's the only way to eat properly.

I'm not saying that you have to prepare major meals—you can use protein shakes, too. I've been fortunate to work for MET-Rx for the past seven years, and I actually use the products I endorse on a daily basis. How many spokespeople can claim the same? I believe in and use MET-Rx shakes because they fit my eating program perfectly: They're high in protein, low in carbs, and low in fat. These shakes would be perfect for supplementing your diet as well.

I eat three meals and drink two protein shakes every day. RTD, or "ready to drink," shakes are great because you can take them wherever you go, including work and vacations. It would be very time-consuming and expensive if you were to try to eat five meals of food a day, so don't even attempt it.

The TRUTH's Diet-Formula Guidelines

1 gram of protein per current body weight

1 gram of carbohydrates per current body weight

.22 grams of fat x body weight

Let's look at a couple examples so that you can see how easy it is to work with this formula. We'll use a 200-pound person and a 125-pound person as our models.

200-POUND PERSON

Daily protein intake: 200 x 1 = 200 grams of protein per day

Daily carb intake: 200 x 1 = 200 grams of carbs per day

Daily fat intake: 200 x .22 = 44 grams of fat per day

Total calories = 1,996

(*Note:* Carbs and protein = 4 calories per gram, while fat = 9 calories a gram.)

125-POUND PERSON

Daily protein intake: 125 x 1 = 125 grams of protein per day

Daily carb intake: 125 x 1 = 125 grams of carb per day

Daily fat intake: 125 x .22 = 27 (round off) grams of fat per day

Total calories = 1,243

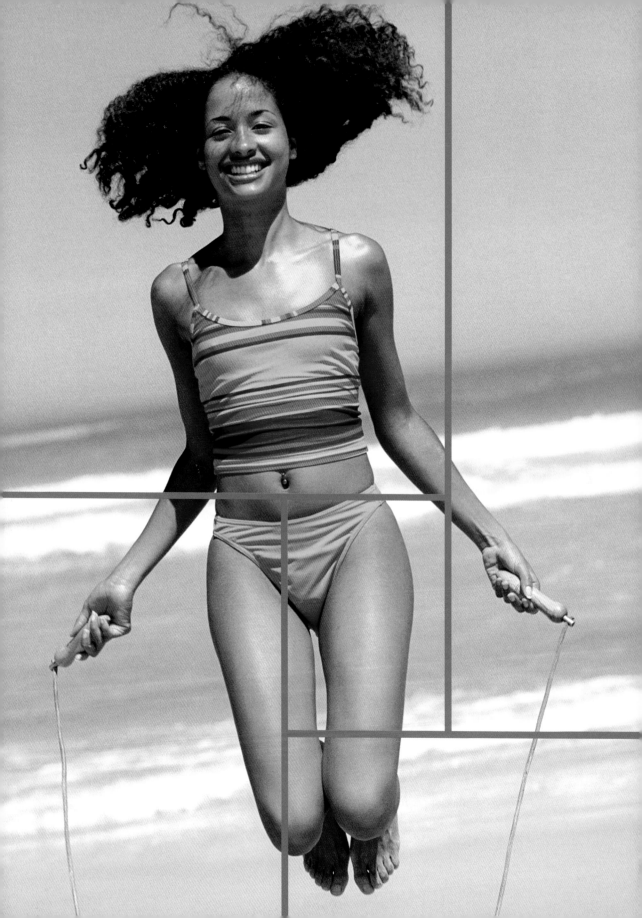

CHAPTER 7

FAT-BURNING AND CARDIO

One of the biggest mistakes people make in their quest for the perfect six-pack is excluding cardiovascular exercise. I wish I could say that if you skip the cardio you'll achieve that flat stomach anyway, but I'd be lying to you—it's absolutely necessary.

I know people who hate cardio and will find any excuse not to do it. In fact, I once had a client tell me that running made his stomach bloated, so he refused to do so. Yet the fact of the matter is that there's no way around it: You need to combine diet, cardio, and weight training for that triple fitness threat.

For the last couple months, I've jotted down any question that a client asks me about cardio, and I came up with the top 15 questions about the thing we dread the most. (Come on—it's not *that* bad!)

Question #1: "Why do I have to do cardio if I'm only trying to achieve a flat stomach?"

Frank says: The most effective way to permanently lose weight is to combine cardio, strength training, and a healthy diet. If you're trying to achieve a trim midsection, then you've got to lose *body fat,* not just weight. Cardio will help you do so by burning excess calories, which will hopefully reduce your body fat if you're also following the right eating program. Cardio allows you to keep your weight under control as well.

Question #2: "Are there any other benefits of cardio?"

Frank says: I could write an entire book about the wonders of cardiovascular exercise, but for now, here are my top five reasons why you should do it (besides the fact it helps you burn calories and fat):

1. It reduces your risk of a heart attack.
2. It helps lower your blood pressure.
3. It naturally boosts your metabolism.
4. It alleviates stress.
5. It increases your energy for sex and enhances lung capacity.

Now I think those are some pretty good reasons to make cardio a regular, everyday thing.

Question #3: "When's the best time to do cardio?"

Frank says: First thing in the morning on an empty stomach. When I say "empty stomach," I mean that you shouldn't even have a glass of orange juice. Whatever form you choose—Rollerblading, jogging, biking, or jumping rope—the morning is the best time to do cardio. That's because you haven't eaten anything in the past six to eight hours (or however long you slept). When the body finds that there aren't any carbs to burn, it will go directly to stored body fat. If you choose to do cardio later in the day after a few meals, all you'll be burning off are those calories you've just eaten. In other words, cardio on an empty stomach burns body fat, while cardio after you've eaten burns calories and carbs.

Question #4: "If I'm going to do your ab and weight-training program, should I do cardio before or after my workout?"

Frank says: Different studies show different things, but I'd do my weight-training and ab routine before I did my cardiovascular exercise because strength training depletes the glycogen in the body as a primary source of energy. Cardio after weight training will result in your body burning up fat as an energy source because you've already depleted your glycogen levels with the weight-training workout. Cardio will also help with the removal of lactic acid, which builds up after weight training.

Question #5: "Should I stretch before I do my cardio routine?"

Frank says: Actually, you should do a light warm-up before you stretch. Cold muscles tear, so it's important that you follow through and do a 5- to 10-minute warm-up. Then a full-body stretch will do wonders for your body, as it will reduce the physical stress you'll be putting on your muscles when you work out. Tight muscles are tense muscles, and muscle tension saps your body of energy—which isn't exactly the best way to get those abs of steel.

Question #6: "What does 'RHR' stand for?"

Frank says: I know that when we trainers talk, it sometimes sounds as if we're ER doctors, but it's not really that complicated. RHR means *resting heart rate,* or the number of times your heart beats per minute when your body is at rest. You can find out your RHR very easily. First, make sure that you're completely relaxed, and place two fingers on the side of your neck to find your pulse. Next, count the number of beats you feel in a minute's time. The average RHR for a man is 70 bpm (beats per minute) while the average RHR for a woman is 75 bpm. (People who work out regularly and athletes who are in peak physical condition will have a lower RHR because it takes less effort and fewer beats per minute for their hearts to pump blood through their bodies.) By knowing your RHR, you can gauge your workouts more efficiently and measure your improvements more precisely.

Question #7: "What do 'MHR' and 'THR' stand for?"

Frank says: MHR stands for *maximum heart rate,* or the maximum amount of beats your heart pumps in a minute. When you do cardiovascular exercise, it's important to do so at the right levels, so you might find yourself asking the following questions: *Should I be moving faster? How long should I be going this fast? How do I know if I'm overdoing it?* This is where heart-rate-zone training comes in.

By following the equation below, you can find the correct zone to train in:

MHR for women = 226 - your age

MHR for men = 220 - your age

Example: If you're a 30-year-old man, the equation would be 220 - 30 = 190

THR means *target heart rate.* The equation for figuring out your target heart-rate range is: MHR x 0.55 (55%) to MHR x .90 (90%). Or based on the 30-year-old above, it would be from 190 x .55 to 190 x .90, or 104.5 to 171. That means that this guy's target rate would be between 104.5 and 171 bpm.

Question #8: "What's the difference between the various heart-rate ranges?"

Frank says: If you're a beginner, you should stay within 55%–60% of your MHR; but if your goal is to lose body fat, then you need to be within 60–70% of your MHR (this is also known as the weight-management zone). Working out at 70–80% of your maximum heart rate will help improve your endurance, plus improve function of your lungs, heart, and respiratory rate; while working out at 80–90% will further help endurance and increase speed, but shouldn't be done without supervision.

Exercising at 90% of your MHR is the *anaerobic range,* which should only be done in short bursts. This range is so intense that your cardiovascular system can't get oxygen to the muscles, and it's commonly used in interval-training routines to help performance. Be very careful— if you train in this range, you can easily get hurt.

The chart below easily illustrates the right MHR broken down by age groups:

AGE	50% MHR	60% MHR	70% MHR	80% MHR
18–25	99	119	139	159
26–30	95	115	134	153
31–36	93	112	130	149
37–42	90	108	126	144
43–50	86	103	121	138
51–58	83	99	116	133
59–65	79	95	110	126
65+	76	91	106	121

Question #9: "I always see people in the gym wearing heart-rate monitors. Should I get one?"

Frank says: A heart-rate monitor (HRM) makes life a lot easier, especially for those of you who are just starting out. Perhaps you've stood on a treadmill and were baffled when asked to punch in your speed and workout level. You had no idea, so you pushed a few buttons and just started walking. This is one of the reasons why you should definitely purchase an HRM. It's like having your own personal trainer who tells you when to slow down or speed up. Since it will figure out your 60–70% target zone, you'll know whether or not you should increase the speed or level on the treadmill. An HRM makes your workout much more effective and safe, since you'll get the most out of every training session.

If you want to reach your fitness goals, then you have to exercise in the correct zone. An HRM is the most accurate way to continually measure your heart rate and ensure that you're working out at the right intensity level. Besides being crucial to your performance, this device will let you know how the most important muscle in your body is doing—and it will let you know if you're overdoing it or when you've fully recovered during interval training. A heart-rate monitor is necessary for everyone and anyone who steps into the gym because it's one of the most reliable indicators of your fitness level.

Question #10: "How often—and for how long—should I do cardio for?"

Frank says: It all depends on your level of fitness. If you're just starting out, no one would expect you to go for it six days a week for an hour a session. And if your only form of exercise is getting off the couch and answering the door to get your pizza, then *anything* you do is going to help. Seriously, if you haven't done any cardio in the last year, then it's best to build your sessions up gradually. I suggest that you walk for 15 minutes three days a week, and try to keep your MHR at 60%. After a few sessions, if you feel as if you're ready to increase your duration, then add 5 minutes to your session. The goal is to be able to make cardiovascular exercise a regular part of your life.

For those of you who aren't beginners, there's no definitive plan to follow here. Everyone's body reacts differently to the amount and frequency of cardio they do, but I suggest that for general fitness, you should exercise between three to five days a week for 20–30 minutes. For fat burning, I've found that the best results come from alternating high and low intensity cardio, four to six days a week, for 20–60 minutes. Obviously, you'd do the high-intensity cardio for a lesser time (20 minutes).

Also, keep in mind that cardio works in conjunction with your diet program, so if you're eating 500 calories more a day than you're burning, then you're still going to gain weight no matter how much cardio you're doing. Let's do some simple math: If you eat 500 calories a day more then you burn, it will add up to 3,500 calories by the end of the week, which translates into a one-pound weight gain. Sorry to break the bad news to you.

Question #11: "I've heard that bodybuilders sometimes do cardio more than once a day. Is this too much?"

Frank says: Bodybuilders are notorious for this. After all, the goal of any bodybuilder who's training for a competition is to get his or her body fat down to the lowest possible percentage. The way he or she accomplishes this is by following a very strict precontest diet, training daily with weights, and doing lots of cardio. Bodybuilders eat a lot of food when they're in pre-contest mode, because they're trying to build lean muscle as they're losing body fat. In order to do so, they do cardio twice a day, including once in the morning on an empty stomach when their glycogen levels are at the lowest (burning stored fat), and once again after their weight-training workout when their glycogen levels are depleted to burn even more fat.

Doing cardio twice a day is effective if it's for a short period of time—if you do it for a long period, then you're going to feel the ill effects of overtraining, including flulike symptoms, muscle atrophy, and diarrhea, to name a few. The plan of twice-a-day cardio is used by a lot of people who want to lose weight or build up their endurance quickly; and many actors and actresses who need to get in shape for a movie fast are likely to use this kind of workout scheme. If you're planning on doing cardio twice a day, then do it for a *short period of time* or for only a few days a week. If you do it too much and for too long, it will be counterproductive.

Question #12: "Which is better: long-duration cardio or short, intense sessions?"

Frank says: I've tried both low-intensity, long-duration (LILD) and high-intensity, short-duration (HISD) exercise, and they're both beneficial. Some people get bored doing 60 minutes of cardio per session, so they prefer a 20-minute high-impact session. Others' bodies get injured when following HISD—their muscles get pulled and strained when they push that far—so they like the slower pace of LILD. It all depends on what you enjoy doing. I believe that if you're looking for a great way to improve your cardiovascular fitness, then your program should include a combination of both LILD and HISD.

Question #13: "Should I vary my form of cardio?"

Frank says: When people talk about doing cardio, it always conjures up visions of someone jogging on the treadmill every day. Boring, boring, boring! It's important to find other activities that are enjoyable as well as being effective. Doing cardio doesn't mean that you're chained to one machine for life. You should try all your gym has to offer—the treadmill, stepper, elliptical rider, bicycle, and even aerobic classes. Variety is the spice of life, so spice up your cardio routines by trying different things.

When you get sick of looking at the red numbers on the indoor machines' screens, simply go outside and have some fun. It's a known fact that people who do a fitness activity they love rather than something they hate are much more successful at sticking to it. So get out there and swim, Rollerblade, play tennis, and have some fun while you burn calories.

Question #14: "What types of cardio activities burn the most calories?"

Frank says: The amount of calories you'll burn is based upon your weight, the cardio activity you're going to do, and how intensely you perform that activity. The more intensely you work, the more calories you're going to burn.

Below, you'll notice that I've provided you with a variety of activities that you can follow, along with how many calories you'll burn in a 10-minute time frame doing them. This table lists a variety of exercises and the caloric expenditures for a 123-pound woman and a 170-pound man. (Data for this table was taken from *Reebok Instructor News,* Volume 5, Number 2, 1997.)

ACTIVITY AND CALORIES/ 10 MINS.	123-LB. WOMAN	170-LB. MAN
Basketball	77	106
Cycling (5.5 mph)	36	49
Cycling (9.4 mph)	56	74
Cycling (racing)	95	130
Dance exercise (high-impact aerobics)	94	124
Dance exercise (low-impact aerobics)	80	105
Football	74	102
Racquetball	76	107
Rope skipping (slow)	82	116

Rope skipping (fast)	100	142
Running (8 mins./mile)	113	150
Running (11½ mins./mile)	76	100
Skiing (cross country)	80	106
Soccer	78	107
StairMaster	88	122
Step aerobics (4-inch bench)	48	66
Step aerobics (6-inch bench)	58	80
Step aerobics (8-inch bench)	67	92
Step aerobics (10-inch bench)	75	104
Swimming (backstroke)	95	130
Swimming (breaststroke)	91	125
Swimming (fast crawl)	87	120
Swimming (slow crawl)	95	130
Swimming (sidestroke)	68	90
Swimming (treading water)	35	48
Tennis (singles)	61	81
Volleyball	28	39
Weight training (super circuit)	104	137
Weight training (muscular strength)	44	60
Weight training (muscular endurance)	58	80
Walking (3.5 mph)	45	59

Question #15: "Should I cool down after my cardio workout? And is it really that important to stretch?"

Frank says: Don't just abruptly jump off the treadmill—you need to cool down to physically and mentally recover. You also want to give your heart a chance to return to its resting rate without shocking it; after all, you don't want it to work overtime to return to normal. So it's best to take 5 minutes to wind down and reflect on what you've just accomplished, clear your head, and finish the workout in a positive frame of mind.

And you absolutely must stretch to enhance your muscle strength and flexibility. I suggest doing a 5- to 10-minute full-body stretch after your cardio session.

Last Words on Cardio

I hope that this chapter has opened your eyes and made you realize how important cardio is when it comes to obtaining that flat, ripped midsection. Unless you're a genetic marvel, there's no chance of achieving the perfect six-pack without cardiovascular exercise. If you add cardio to your daily life, it will create a healthier you, while increasing your chances of obtaining the abs you always wanted. Just remember that Rome wasn't built in a day—and you won't be either—so pace yourself and train smart, and you'll be rewarded in the form of a healthier and leaner you.

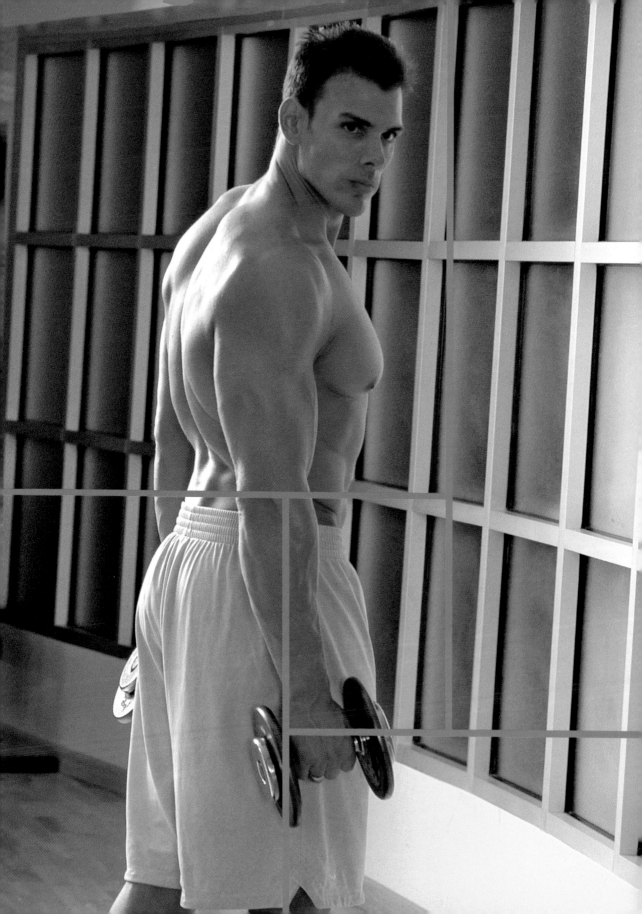

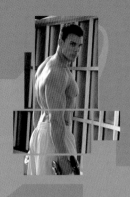

CHAPTER 8

AB-RACADABRA: ALL YOUR AB QUESTIONS ANSWERED

Now I'd like to cut through all the scientific mumbo jumbo that usually occurs when fitness experts explain how you're supposed to build your abs. (I liked the last chapter so much that I decided to repeat the question-and-answer format here.)

Question: "What other benefits besides looking good will I get out of training my midsection?"

Frank says: Well, let's not forget that when you're trying to achieve a ripped set of abs, you're also losing body fat, thus reducing your risk of cardiovascular disease, stroke, hypertension, and certain types of cancer as well. And when you train your abdominal muscles, you're also helping to support your lower back and improve your posture.

How many Americans suffer from lower back pain, and how many of them are out of shape? A sturdy and functional core (which consists of the rectus abdominis, transverse abdominis, internal and external obliques, hip flexors, and the lower back or *erector spinae*) will help you keep your lower back healthy and improve the ease with which you do everyday activities. Also, keep in mind that if you're an athlete, strong abs and back muscles are crucial to your performance in the gym and on the playing field. There isn't one sport you can do where a strong core won't make a difference. So there's much more to abs then oiling up your six-pack for the beach.

Question: "What's the proper way to breathe during an ab exercise?"

Frank says: Let me start off by saying that no matter what you do, you should never hold your breath during the exercise. If you do (like so many people I see), you can pass out or possibly have a stroke. I also suggest that you breathe throughout the exercise, exhaling on the upward portions and inhaling on the downward ones. If this gives you trouble, then breathe naturally. But for God's sake, *don't hold your breath.*

Question: "Can anyone build a great set of abs?"

Frank says: No. There's one type of person who is unable to have a washboard stomach, and that's a lazy person. But other than that, anyone can have a set of defined abs if they follow the guidelines of training and nutrition I've laid out in this book.

The speed with which you'll obtain a toned midsection will be based on a few factors, including your current physical condition. If you're 50 pounds overweight and have never been in a gym before, then don't expect an overnight miracle. It will take time. Another component is genetics: Some people respond more quickly than others to a fitness program—that's just the way it is. You can take two people with the same weight, height, and body fat and put them on the same exact program, and you'll always end up with one person who achieves better results. However, they've both changed for the better.

Consistency and willpower are also important: If you embrace proper eating and training as a lifestyle instead of a quick fix and stay consistent, the end result will be a healthier you. And the bonus is that you'll also have a great set of abs!

Question: "Should men and women train their midsections differently?"

Frank says: Nope. The same principles apply for both sexes when it comes to abs—there's no specific gender ab program. Women and men have a similar biological ability to develop strength in their middle; however, women won't achieve the same muscular results as men because of hormonal differences. (But you can still do the same exercises.)

Question: "Can you isolate your upper and lower abs with specific exercises?"

Frank says: No matter what exercise you do for upper or lower abs, you'll still be using the rectus abdominis, which brings about forward torso flexion by stimulating all the muscle fibers as a whole. In other words, you can't specifically isolate a certain part of your abs.

Now, you may be thinking, *Then why are most ab exercises—including the ones in this book—broken down into upper, lower, and obliques?* Well, it's true that you can emphasize certain areas of abs more than others. For example, you'll feel your obliques more if you do a twisting crunch instead of a standard crunch—because even though you're not isolating the obliques and are working other parts of your abs, you're still putting more emphasis on that muscle area with the twisting crunch.

Question: "Is there a specific order in which I should work on my abs?"

Frank says: There are many different opinions on this subject. Personally, I've trained my abs in all different ways in all different sequences, and as long as I did my best, I got a great workout—order and sequence didn't matter. You really have to experiment for yourself to find what order your muscles respond to best. It took me a long time to find out what exercises work best for me, and in what order.

I suggest that if you're just starting out, it's easier to do lower abs first, followed by obliques and then upper abs. This is a great way to structure your ab routine at any level because, like most people, your lower abs are probably weaker—so doing them first in your routine, when you're mentally and physically freshest, is a good idea. Also remember that even when you're working your lower abs, you're engaging your uppers as well. So, when you do an exercise that emphasizes the upper abs last in your routine, they'll already be "pre-exhausted" (or previously worked and fatigued) from doing both the lower and oblique exercises.

I'm a firm believer in not doing the same sequence over and over; otherwise, your abs will adapt and become ineffective. I suggest that you switch the structure and exercises every couple of workouts so that your body doesn't adapt to the program. Variety is important.

Question: "Can I train my abs every day?"

Frank says: I wouldn't train *any* muscle seven days a week. Muscles need time to repair and recuperate, and I believe that ab frequency should be determined by that individual's body type and goals. I will say this, however: Even though the abs are muscles, they can be trained more frequently than others because they rarely fatigue to the point that you'd need an extra day or two to recover. I suggest that you train your abs a minimum of twice a week and a maximum of four. If you're just starting out, twice a week should be fine; and if you're advanced, every other day (or four times a week) is more than enough.

Question: "How many reps and sets should I do?"

Frank says: That will be based on your current level of fitness and what your goals are. In this book, I'll give you many different routines to choose from that will help you achieve your goals. Just remember that abs are muscles and muscles respond both to high reps and low reps and added resistance—so there's more than one right way to train them.

Question: "Should I add some weights or extra resistance to my ab exercises?"

Frank says: Variety is the key to building a perfect six-pack. I think it's a great idea to add some resistance to your workout, which will help stimulate the muscles more and make them stronger.

Question: "How much time during a workout should I devote to training my abs?"

Frank says: Take your time here. I've seen so many people just train as fast as humanly possible, just so they can finish up quickly and go home—but if you really want to make the most of your abdominal workout, then you'll slow down and really focus on what you're doing. Every rep should be done deliberately, with a 1- to 2-second pause where you contract your abs as hard as you can. You should also be breathing correctly and concentrating mentally on your muscles as you're doing the set. This is the most effective way to do a rep. Now, if you speed through a set, you won't be working your abdominals to the fullest, and your development will be severely affected.

Question: "What's the best exercise for abdominals?"

Frank says: It's all about which one works best for *you:* Your individual body type and genetics play a role in this, and the only way you'll find it out is by a long process of trial and error. You'll have to experiment with many different exercises until you discover the ones that are best for you.

Question: "Can I train my abs before my weight-training workout?"

Frank says: Abs should always be done right at the end of any workout. If you were to train them at the start or even the middle of your regimen, any exercise that comes afterward would be much less effective. You see, abs are fixator muscles in more than 90 percent of all exercises (which means that they help stabilize the muscles doing those other exercises), so you'll wear yourself out if you tackle them first.

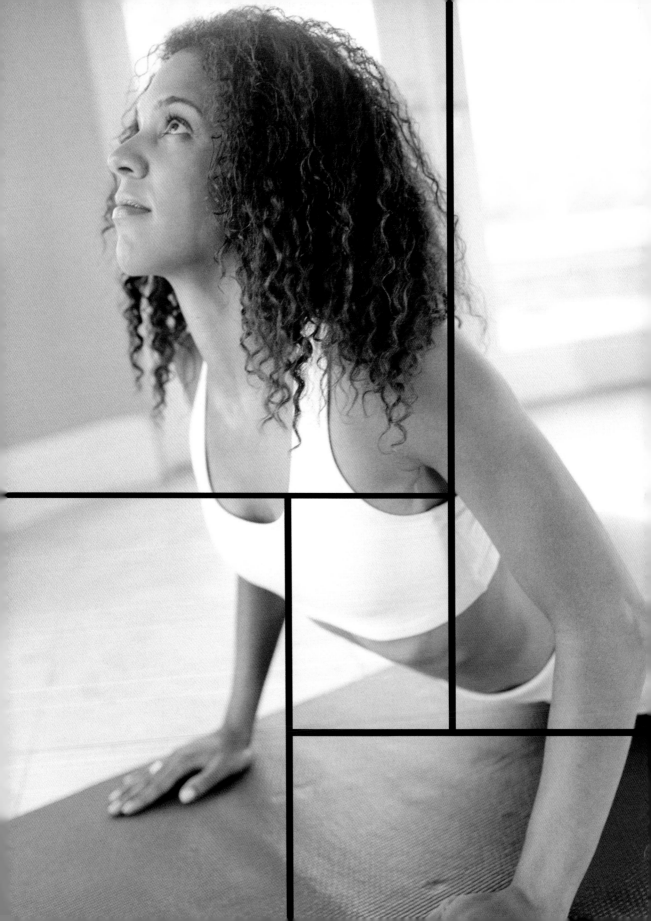

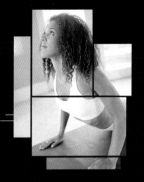

PART III

Hit the Mat

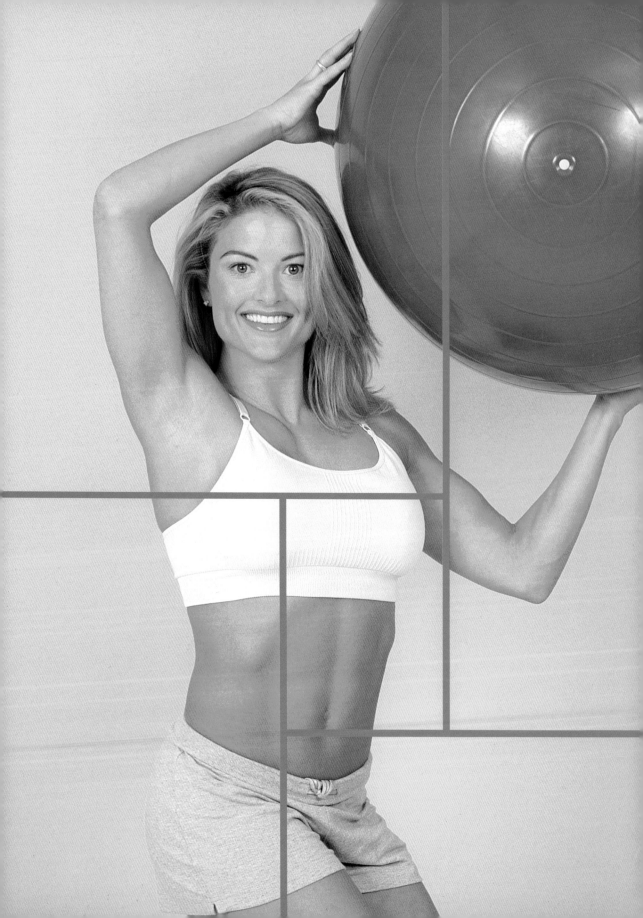

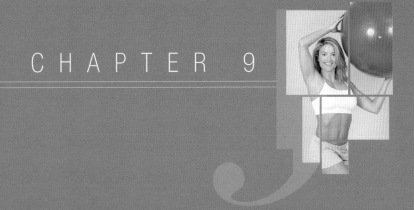

CHAPTER 9

THE BEST AB EXERCISES FOR THE GYM . . . OR ANYWHERE!

It's finally time to start building that six-pack. I'm so proud of you for taking the first step.

In this chapter, I'd like you to keep the following numbers in mind: 15, 5, and 5—15 exercises to do anywhere, 5 you can do with an exercise ball, and 5 to try at the gym. There's something in this chapter for everyone—there are no more excuses for that flabby midesection!

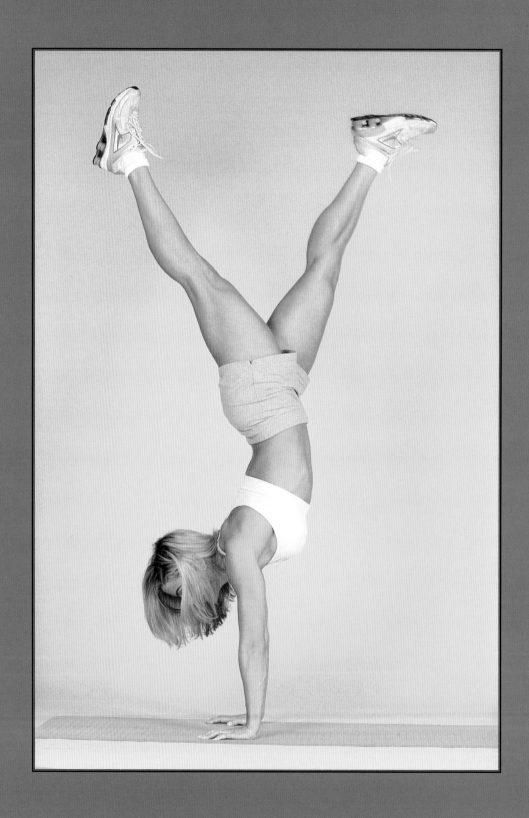

The 15 Best Ab Exercises
You Can Do Anywhere

First, I'd like to give you 15 different exercises that are broken down into categories: upper abs, lower abs, love handles or obliques, and lower back. (This area is included because I expect you to train your lower back during your ab training session.)

You don't need to buy any special equipment, or a gym membership, to do these exercises. The only investment you need to make is your time. Every single one of these exercises can be done at home or outside—just find some comfortable ground, roll out a thick towel, and let's get started.

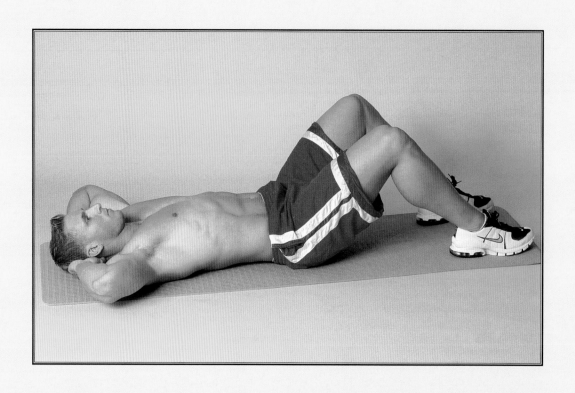

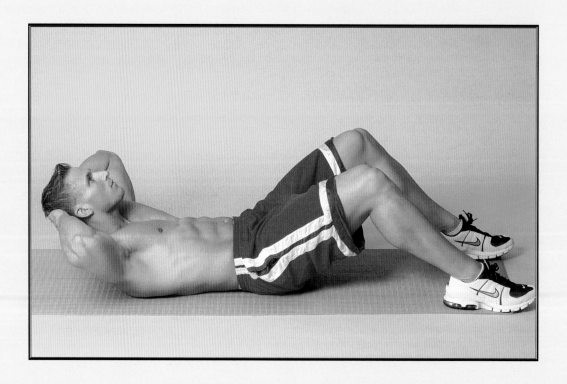

UPPER ABS

Basic Crunch

Lie on your back on a firm, cushioned surface (a carpeted floor or an exercise mat will work fine—a hard surface will be rough on your back), with your knees bent and feet flat. It's up to you: You can either cross your arms comfortably over your chest or lightly hold the back of your neck and then tense your rectus abdominis muscle. Use this muscle alone to lift your upper torso off the floor. Next, contract your abs (for a second or two), and then lower your shoulders back to the starting position. Exhale during the up movement and inhale during the return to the floor. Don't forget to breathe!

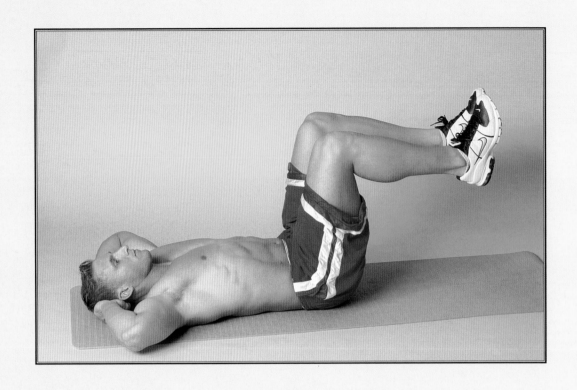

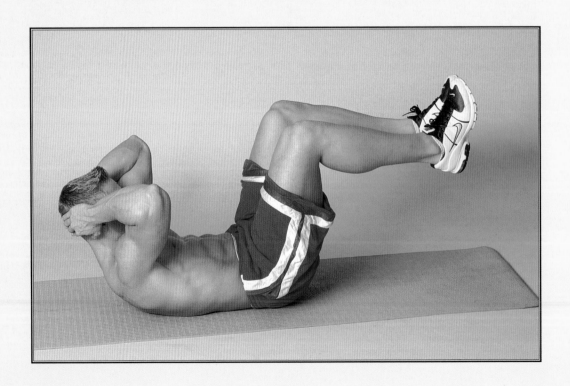

U P P E R   A B S

Crunches—Knees in the Air

Lie on your back and raise your legs so that your thighs are perpendicular to your body, placing your calves and feet parallel to the floor and your hands in the position of your choice. Then tense your rectus abdominis muscle. Use this muscle alone to lift your upper torso off the floor. Next, contract your abs, and then lower your shoulders back to the starting position.

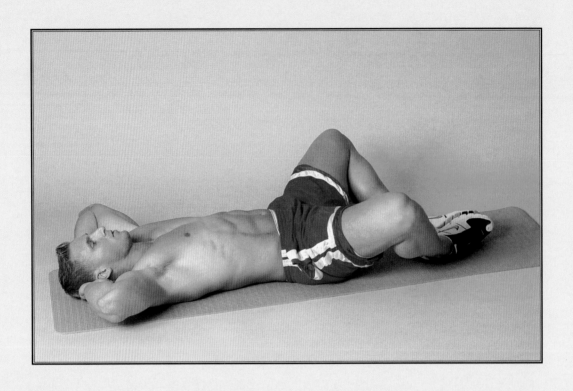

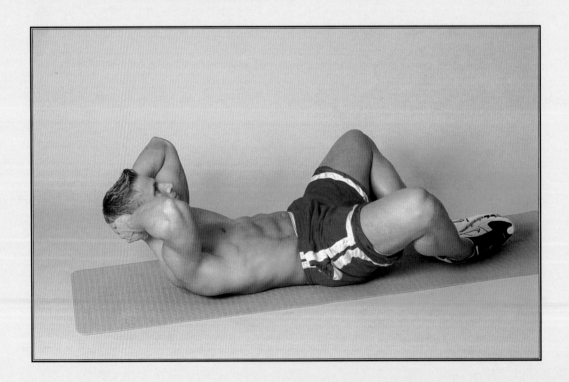

UPPER ABS

Butterfly Crunch

Lie on the floor with your knees bent and the soles of your feet together (your knees should drop out to the side or as far as your flexibility allows), and place your hands in the position of your choice. Next, tense your rectus abdominis muscle. Use this muscle alone to lift your upper torso off the floor. Next, contract your abs, and then lower your shoulders back to the starting position. (See **Crunches—Knees in the Air** on p. 77.)

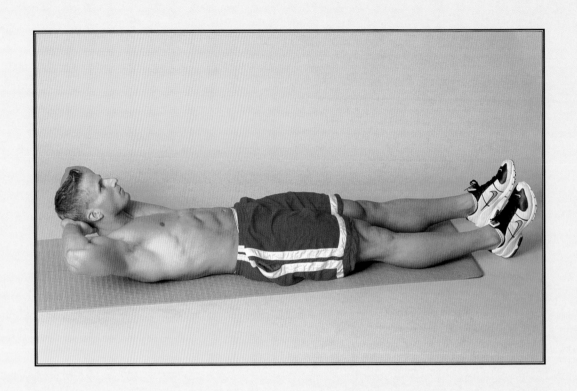

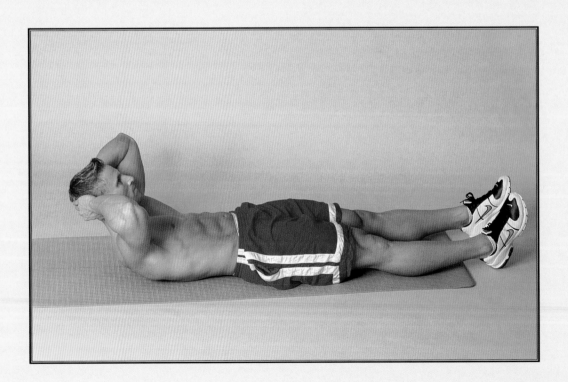

UPPER ABS

Crunches—Legs Straight Out

Lie on your back, legs extended straight out (think of it as lying perfectly straight) with your arms in the position of your choice. Then tense your rectus abdominis muscle. Use this muscle alone to lift your upper torso off the floor. Next, contract your abs, and then lower your shoulders back to the starting position. (See **Crunches—Knees in the Air** on p. 77.)

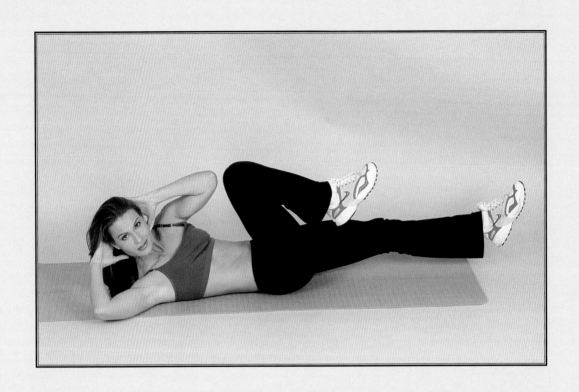

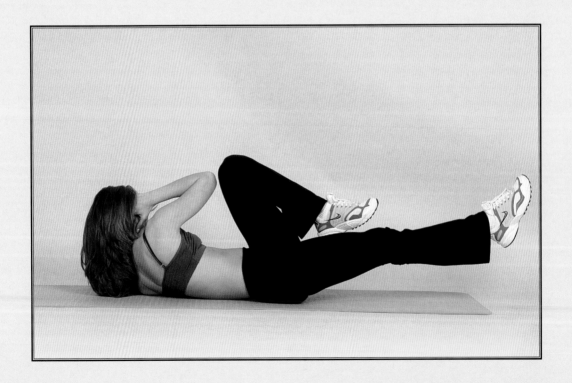

LOWER ABS

Bicycles

Lie faceup on the floor with your hands clasped loosely behind your head for support. Curl your upper back off the floor while pressing your lower back firmly against the floor. While maintaining this basic trunk curl position, lift both legs about 8–12 inches off the floor. Immediately bring your left knee back toward your chest while keeping your right leg straight. Try to touch your right elbow to your left knee by turning your torso to the left. Now reverse your leg positions, simultaneously pushing your left leg forward to full knee extension and pulling your right leg backward to full knee flexion. Try to touch your left elbow to your right knee by turning your torso to the right.

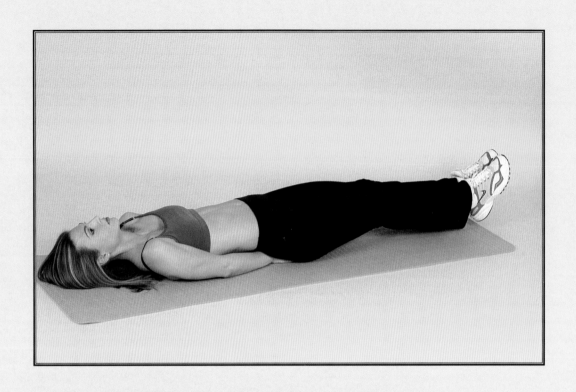

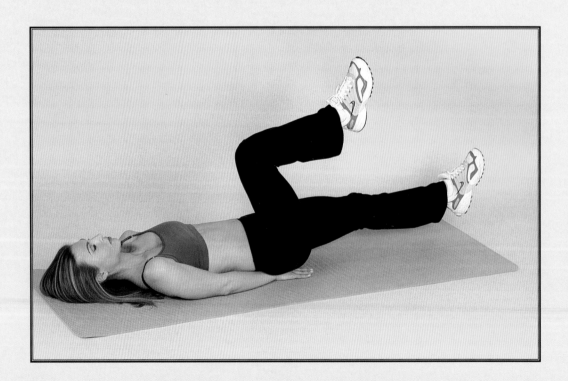

LOWER ABS

Alternate Knee Tucks

Lie on your back, supporting yourself on your elbows and keeping your hands under your buttocks/hips for support. Lift both legs clear up off the floor: Bring one knee up as close to your shoulder as possible, then straighten that leg back out while simultaneously bringing the other knee up to the shoulder. Continue this movement with both legs moving at the same time— one up and one down. (Your legs should be off the floor throughout the exercise.)

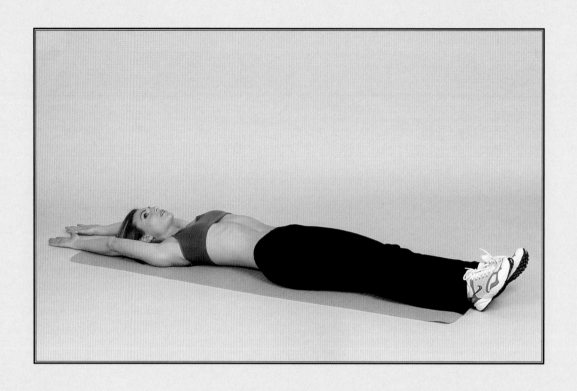

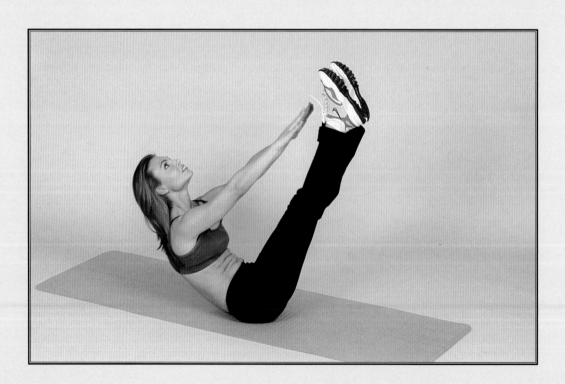

LOWER ABS

Toe-Touch Crunches

Lie on your back on the floor (choose a comfortable surface) with your arms straight over your head and legs extended straight. Sit up (lift shoulders slightly) by reaching upward with your hands, and try to touch your toes with your fingertips. Pause for a second or two, contract your abs, and then relax. Return to the starting position.

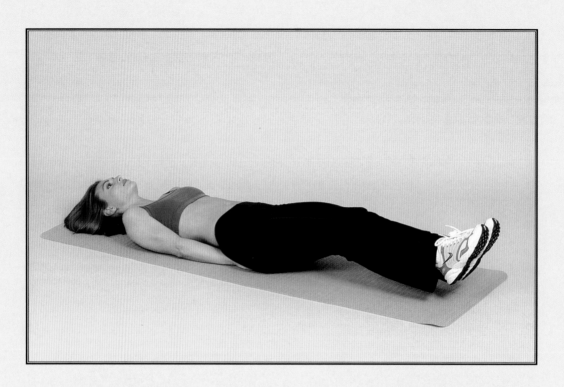

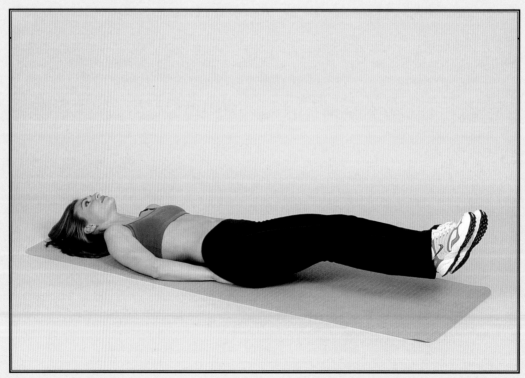

LOWER ABS

Lying Leg Raise (lower)

Lie on your back, legs extended straight out (think of it as lying perfectly straight) with your hands slightly under your buttocks and your palms facing down. This will tilt your pelvis up and the small of your back down. Now, with your knees slightly bent, use your lower abs to raise your feet about 6 inches off the floor. Hold and contract your abs for a count of 1 or 2, and then slowly lower your feet back down.

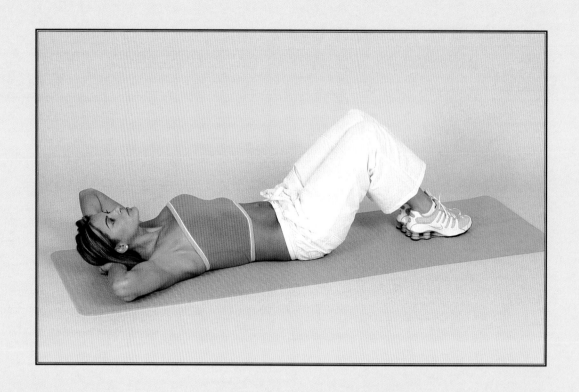

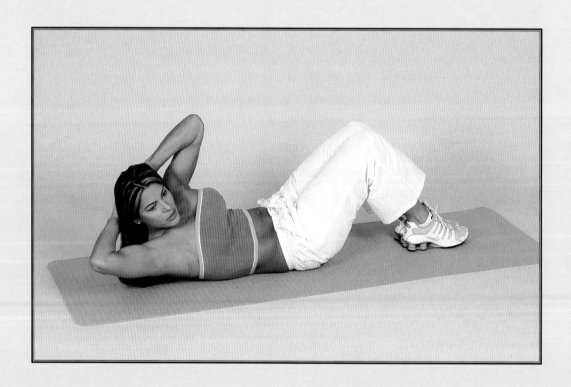

OBLIQUES (LOVE HANDLES)

Cross-Knee Crunch

Lie on your back with your knees bent, feet flat on the ground, and legs together. Your hands should be lightly touching the sides of your head. Now curl your shoulders off the floor, twisting your torso toward your right knee. Contract your abs, and go back to starting position. Curl up again, this time twisting to the left.

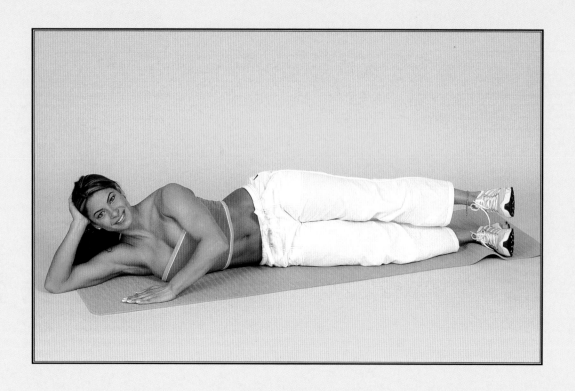

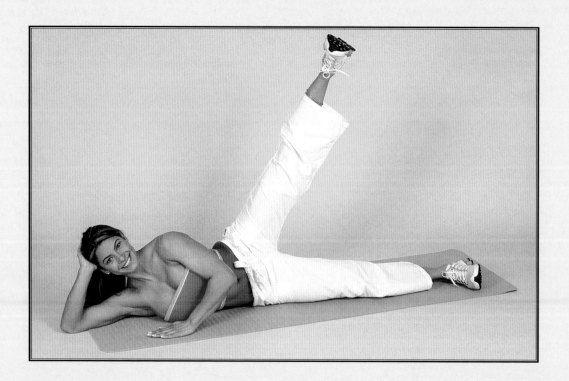

OBLIQUES (LOVE HANDLES)

Single-Side Leg Raise

Lie on your right side and rest your head on your right hand. Place your left hand, palm down, in front of you (to brace your body) and bend your right leg slightly. Your left leg should remain straight and raised a few inches above your right leg. Lift your left leg straight up: Hold for a second or two, then lower. Now repeat the exercise on your left side.

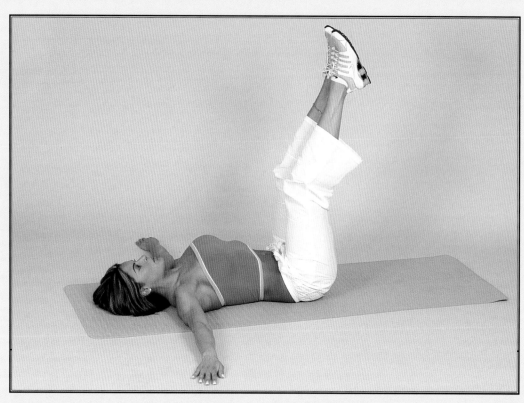

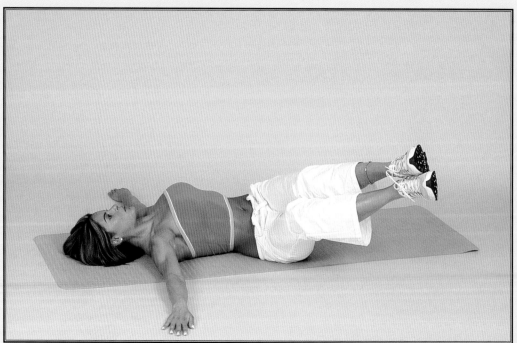

OBLIQUES (LOVE HANDLES)

Double Leg Over

Lie flat on your back with your arms out to your sides, palms facing down. Curl your knees toward your chest, and then extend your legs up toward the sky. Now slowly rotate your pelvis to the right and bring your legs across your body, lowering your feet toward the floor. Rotate back to the center. Change directions, rotating your legs to the left.

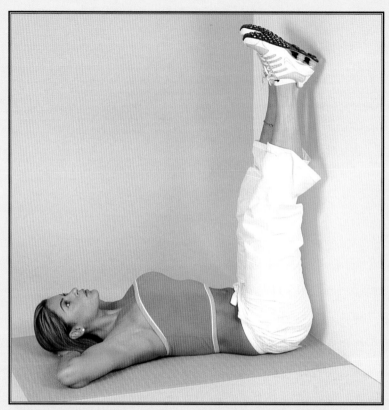

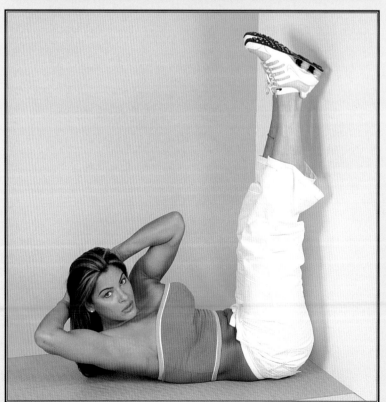

OBLIQUES (LOVE HANDLES)

Twisting Crunch—Feet Against Wall

Lie down next to a wall and place your legs up on it. Make sure that your legs and butt are flat against the wall, with your feet pointing straight up to the sky. Place your hands lightly against the sides of your head, elbows slightly off the floor, then slowly curl your trunk (torso) up off the floor and twist to the left. Repeat, this time twisting to the right side.

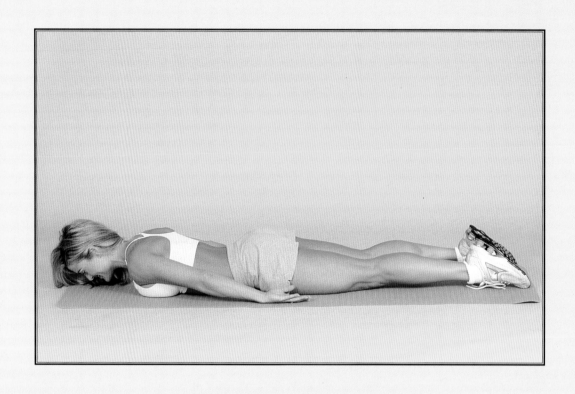

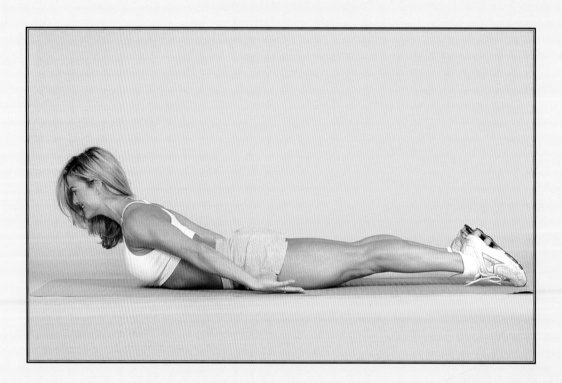

LOWER BACK

Back Extension

Lie on your stomach on a comfortable surface. Place your arms at your sides so that your hands are by your hips. Now, raise your head and shoulders off the mat as high as you can. Hold for a few seconds, then lower your head and shoulders back down to the mat; repeat.

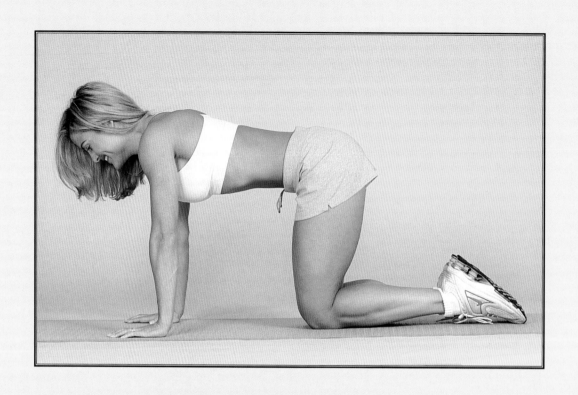

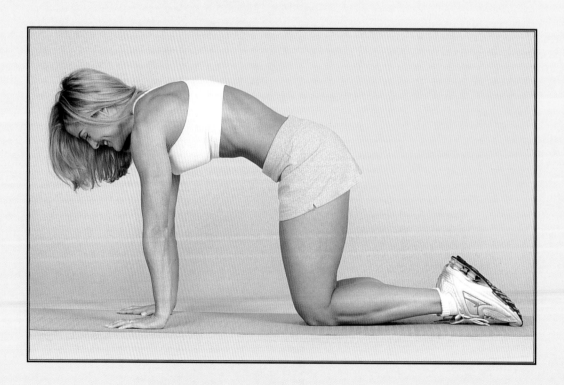

LOWER BACK

Cat and Camel

Get down on all fours with knees and hands on the floor and your back and neck in a neutral, straight position. Next, slowly tighten lower abdominals, rounding the back toward the ceiling. Hold for five seconds; release and return to neutral position. Then arch the back slightly, holding for five seconds; release and return to neutral position.

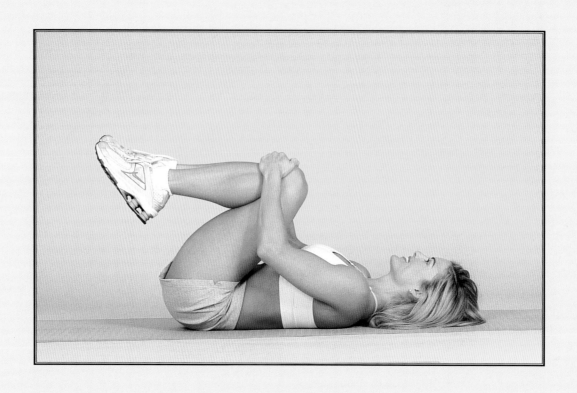

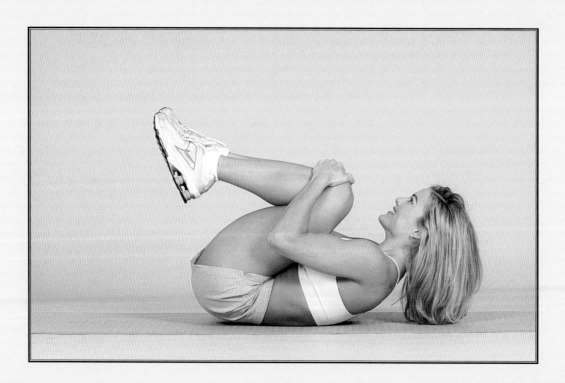

LOWER BACK

Back Flexion

Lie on your back, pulling both knees to your chest while simultaneously flexing your head forward until you reach a comfortable stretch in a balled-up position. Do 5–10 repetitions, holding each one for 5–10 seconds.

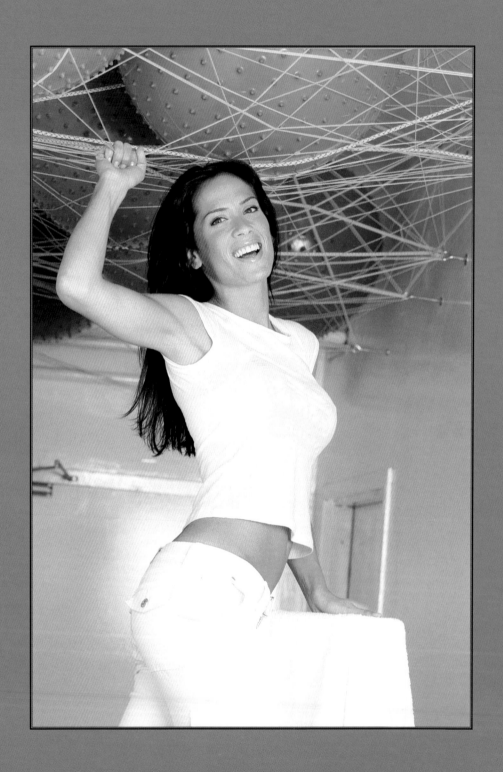

Using an Exercise Ball

Okay, I've given you the 15 no-frills exercises you can do anywhere. Now you're going to have to reach into your pockets and make a little investment. It's a good one, though—for the $20–$40 you'll spend on this item, it will pay you back with a healthier and fitter midsection that you'll have for years. Forget about all those ab machines you see on TV and go buy an exercise or stability ball; after all, they're one of the most versatile pieces of equipment on the market.

There are a number of exercises that you can perform using the ball, and you can pretty much get a whole-body workout with it and a pair of dumbbells. It can be used to develop core body strength, enhance balance, improve posture, and help isolate your abdominals more effectively. I personally like incorporating the ball into my workout because when I do so, it takes a lot of stress off my lower back, and I really feel my abs working when I do a set.

There are dozens of exercise/stability ball exercises out there, but here I'm just going to give you the 5 I've found that work best for my clients and me.

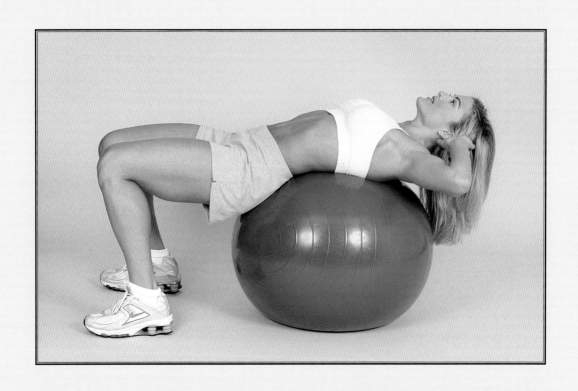

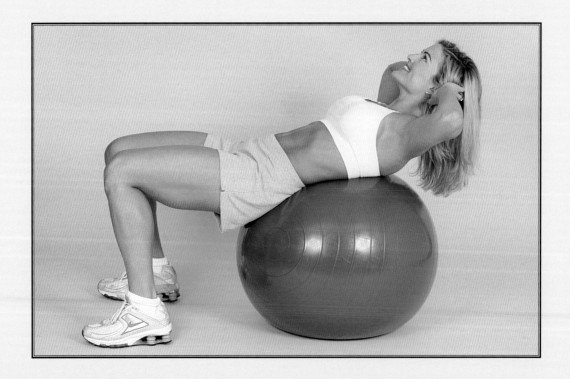

USING AN EXERCISE BALL

Ball Crunch
(Targets upper abs)

Lie on the ball on your back with your feet flat on the floor, your back curved around the ball, and your hands in the position of your choice (behind your head or arms crossed in front). If your neck becomes uncomfortable, place your hands behind your head for support. Slowly curl your trunk, letting your shoulders and upper back lift off the ball. Hold for a second, then return slowly to the starting position. Exhale as you raise your shoulders up off the ball, and inhale as you lower them back down.

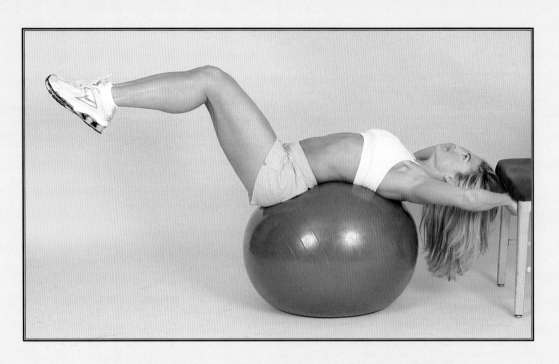

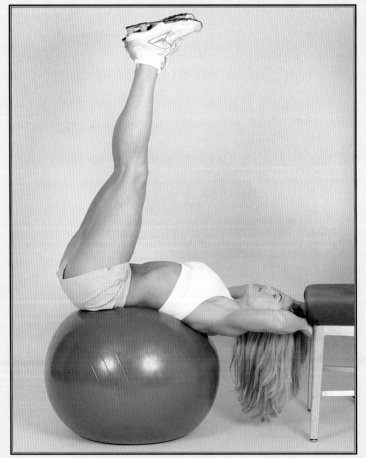

USING AN EXERCISE BALL

Reverse Crunch
(Targets lower abs)

Lie on your back on the ball and reach behind you to grab something sturdy that will support your weight. (A good idea would be a weight bench, a pole, etc.) Bend your hips and knees slightly—your hips should be lower than your shoulders. With your legs extended out in front of you and your knees slightly bent, use just your lower ab muscles to raise your legs and crunch your pelvis toward your rib cage. Hold for a second; then, very slowly and in a controlled motion, lower your legs back to the beginning position.

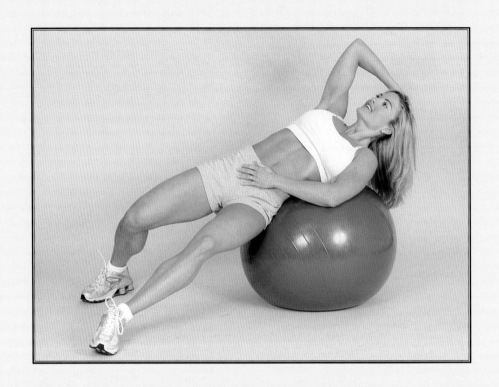

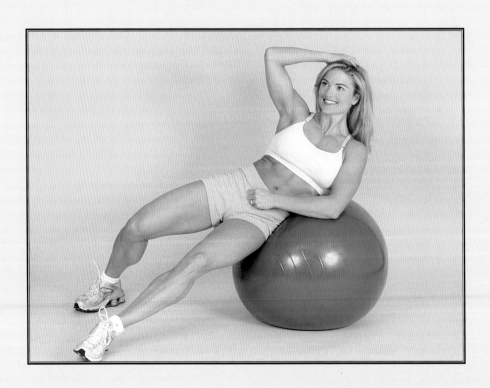

Lying Oblique Crunch
(Targets obliques)

Lie on your left side on the ball, placing your left leg in front, your right leg behind, and your right hand behind your head. Use your right oblique to raise the right side of your rib cage toward the right side of your pelvis. Pause for a second, then slowly lower yourself back to the beginning position. Once you've completed your desired number of reps, switch sides and repeat.

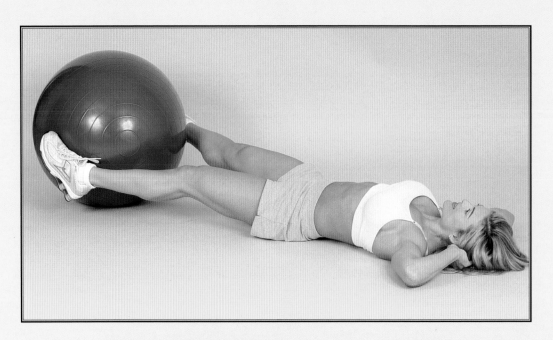

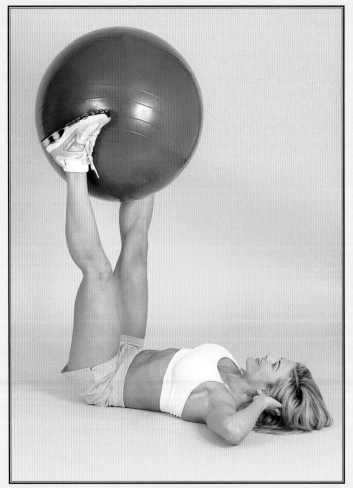

USING AN EXERCISE BALL

Leg Lifts
(Targets lower abs)

Lie flat on your back with your legs fully extended and your hands, palms down, positioned behind your head. Focus on pressing your lower back into the floor. Grasp the ball between your feet and ankles, tighten your abs, and lift your heels a few inches off the floor. Pause for a moment and then lift your legs straight up so that the soles of your feet face the ceiling. Maintain a quick, controlled range of motion as you return to the starting position.

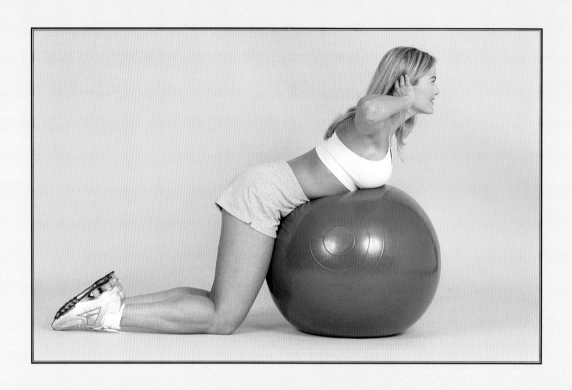

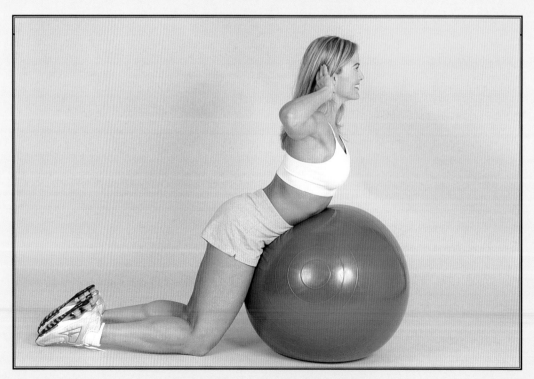

Back Extension

(Targets lower back)

Kneel down in front of the ball and place your belly and rib cage on it. Your upper back should be parallel with the floor while your hands should be placed behind your head, elbows wide. Inhale and use your lower-back muscles to straighten out your upper body. Pause for a second, then go back to the starting position and repeat.

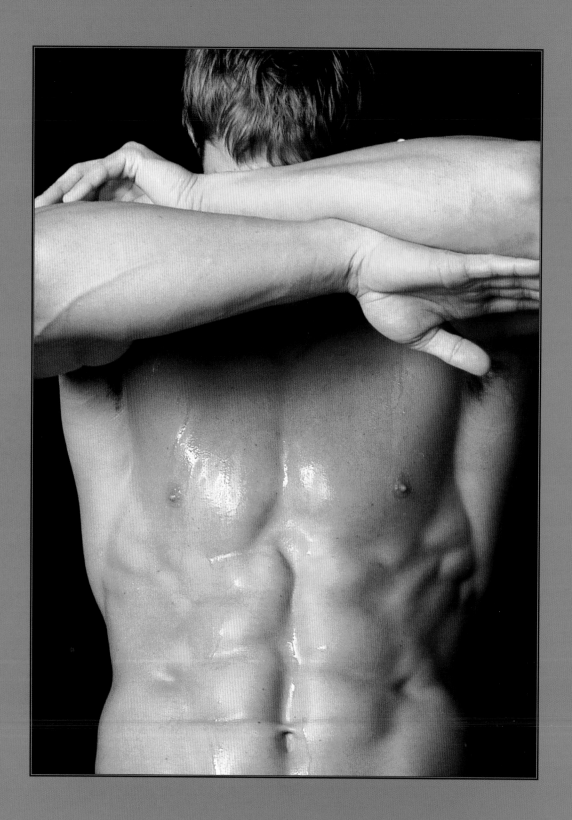

At the Gym

What follows are my 5 favorite ab exercises to do at the gym—in fact, I find them to be the bread and butter of my abdominal program. If you have access to a gym, then I suggest that you include them into your regimen as well.

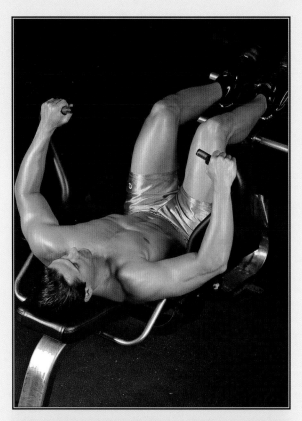

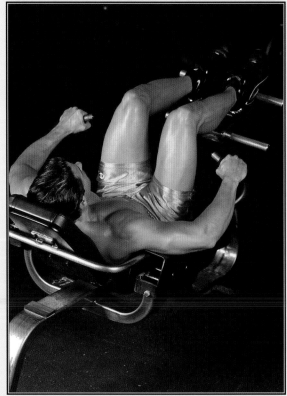

AT THE GYM

Crunch—Machine
(Targets upper and lower abs)

Sit or lie on the machine with your back firmly against the back pad. Lightly grasp the handles and exhale as you curl your shoulders up toward your knees, until your abs are fully contracted. Then inhale as you slowly uncurl to the starting position.

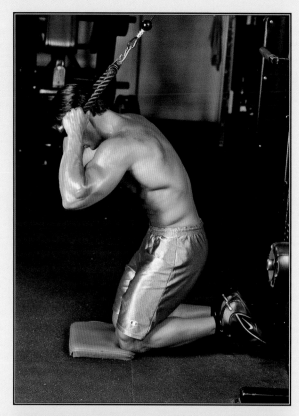

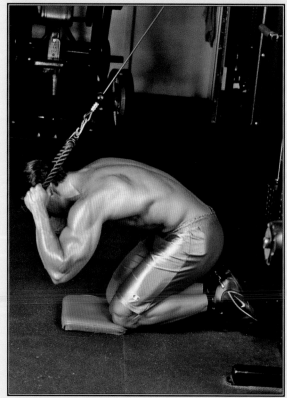

AT THE GYM

Kneeling Crunch—Rope

(Targets upper and lower abs)

Attach a rope to an overhead cable. Facing away from the pulley, grasp the two ends of the rope and pull it down behind you to your ears. Kneel down on the ground to the starting position: sitting upright with your butt resting on your heels. Inhale as you slowly pull down on the rope by curling your torso forward until your abs are fully contracted. Exhale as you slowly straighten up to the starting position.

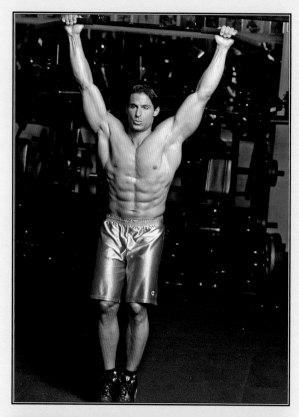

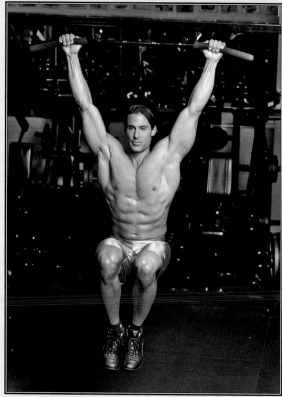

Hanging Reverse Crunch

(Targets lower abs)

Grasp a chin-up bar with your hands shoulder-width apart, palms facing away from you. Hang from the bar with your arms and legs fully extended (your feet shouldn't touch the floor). Maintaining about a 15-degree angle in your knees, inhale as you slowly pull them up to your chest by contracting your abs. Hold this top position for 2 seconds, then exhale as you slowly lower your legs back to the starting position.

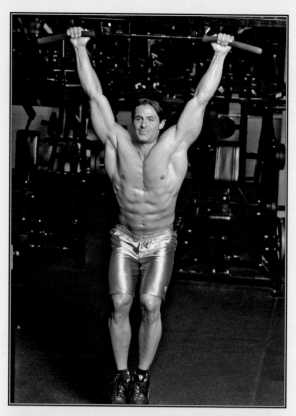

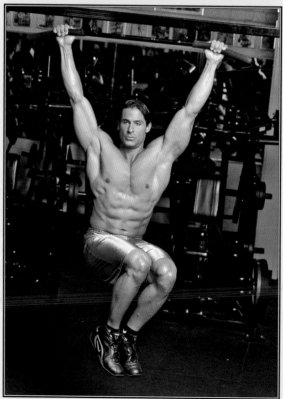

AT THE GYM

Hanging Twisting Leg Raise

(Targets obliques)

Grasp a chin-up bar with your hands shoulder-width apart, palms facing away from you. Hang from the bar with your arms and legs fully extended (your feet shouldn't touch the floor). Inhale as you slowly lift your legs (knees slightly bent) up and to the left. Lift your butt at the top of the motion so that your pelvis tilts toward your abs and contracts them hard. Exhale as you slowly lower your legs back to the starting position. Finish your reps, then repeat the exercise, lifting your legs toward the right.

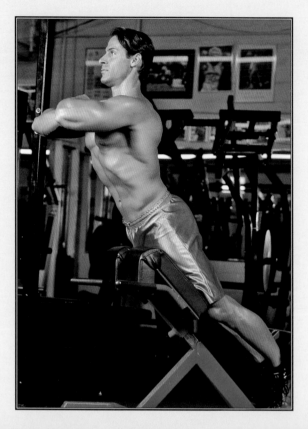

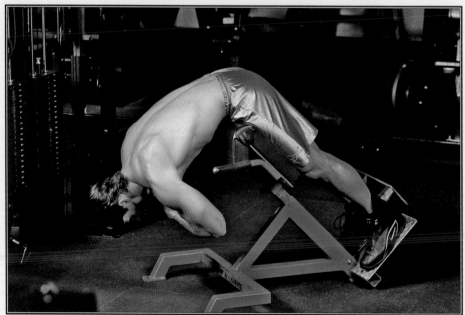

AT THE GYM

Hyperextensions

(Targets lower back)

Lean your pelvis against the pad and place your feet on the footplates, with your heels against the heelpad and your toes pointed forward. Fold your hands across your chest and lean forward. Inhale as you slowly lower your torso forward, bending until your hips form a 60-degree angle. Exhale as you slowly lift your torso back to the starting position.

CHAPTER 10

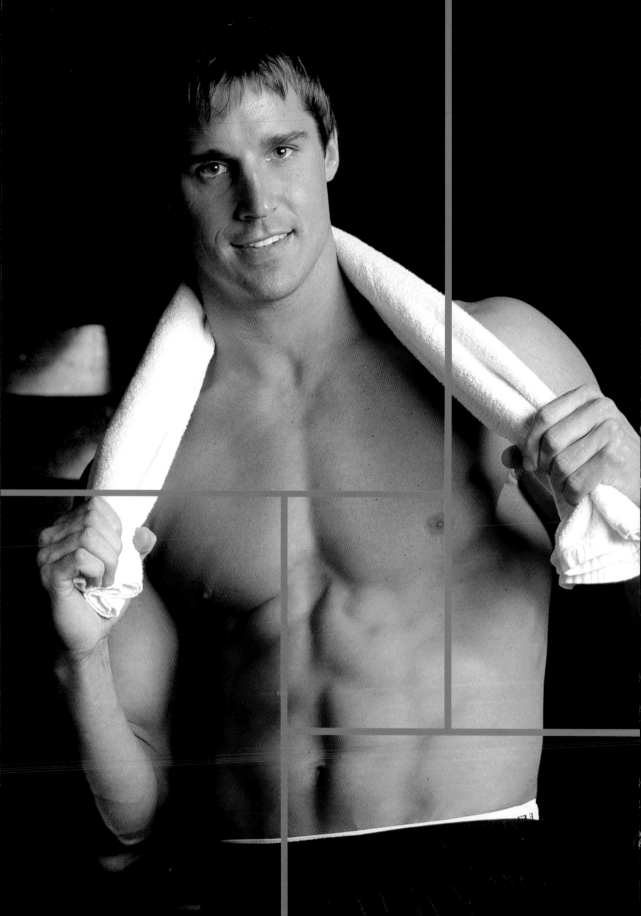

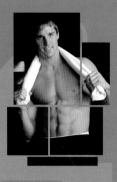

ABDOMINAL ROUTINES

Now that you've familiarized yourself with the 25 exercises I laid out in the previous chapter, I'd like to provide you with some routines in which to use them. But which level—*getting started, beginner, intermediate, or advanced*—should you choose?

Well, if you're just starting out, then you'll want to stick to the basics until your body gets acclimated to the daily grind of working out. It's important that you don't try to progress too fast, or you'll get hurt—so take your time here. Then, when you legitimately feel that you're ready to move on, you can try a more difficult workout.

However, if you've been training for a while and can handle a more advanced workout, there are numerous techniques here that can help take your ab exercises to the next level. But whether you're a beginner or a seasoned veteran, make sure that you're using proper form, are breathing correctly, and are making that mind-muscle connection with every rep.

I have a simple formula that I have my clients follow (and I do as well). It's the formula for success:

CONSISTENCY + INTENSITY = RESULTS

If you follow that equation when it comes to training, and adhere to the rest of the program laid out in this book, then you're definitely going to have the abs of your dreams.

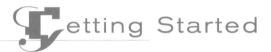etting Started

What's the difference between someone who's just getting started and a beginner? In my mind, the total newbie has never worked out before—ever—so they're probably not in the best physical shape. Now, I know a lot of other books just give you the beginner, intermediate, and advanced levels, but my years as a trainer have taught me that there are some people out there who really have to start from ground zero. There's nothing wrong with that because everyone has to start somewhere. And after all, you can only get better!

If you're just getting started and this is going to be the first ab routine you've ever done, take it easy. Don't let your ego dictate what you should be doing; that is, don't worry about what anyone else is doing—instead, concentrate on the routine you have in front of you. You're just starting out, and you'll have plenty of time to pass up everyone else in the gym.

Just be careful and have fun!

GETTING-STARTED ROUTINE (OR LEVEL 1)

Frequency: 2 times a week—wait 48 hours between ab workouts.

EXERCISE	SETS	REPS	REST BETWEEN SETS
Lying Leg Raise (lower)	2	10–12	40 seconds
Cross-Knee Crunch (obliques)	2	10–12	40 seconds
Basic Crunch (upper)	1	10–12	40 seconds
Back Extension (lower back)	1	10–12	40 seconds

All the exercises for this program were chosen from the 15 Best Ab Exercises You Can Do Anywhere list in the last chapter—after all, if you're just starting out, there's a good chance that you might not have access to a gym. But rest assured that all these exercises are just as good as any ab machine, and they won't slow your progress down one bit.

Yesterday, I used the same exercise sequence in my own ab workout. Remember that I stated earlier in the book that it doesn't matter when it comes to the order of the exercises. However, I believe that most people have weaker lower abs, which is why we'll do those exercises first for now. As you progress, you'll know how your body responds to certain exercises and sequences, so you can change the routine around to benefit your individual needs. (To start, however, please follow the sequences just as I've laid them out for you.)

When Should You Progress to the Next Level?

This depends on you, as everyone progresses at different speeds. Some of you will start at the beginning and move to the next level after just two workouts, but it's fine if you need several sessions before you feel ready to advance. The rule is that if you easily complete the first routine and you've done it at least four times, then it's time to move on. But be honest with yourself before you do so.

Ask yourself the following questions: "Did I use good form and not make use of my body's momentum while completing my reps? Did I do every exercise on the list? Am I physically and mentally ready for my next challenge?" If you answered yes to all three questions, then you're ready to "graduate."

For the Beginner

You'll notice that the beginner's level is more difficult than the previous one—that's because they're two separate categories! I suggest that you follow this routine as written and don't change any of the exercises, since it's very important that you get used to the following routine before you move on. I also want you to keep the lower-back exercise in your routine. When you progress to the next level, you can then decide if you want to keep your back exercises with abs or do them on a separate day. (All the exercises in the chart are from the list of 15 Best Ab Exercises You Can Do Anywhere from the last chapter.)

BEGINNER ROUTINE
(OR LEVEL 2)

Frequency: 2 times a week—wait 48 hours between ab workouts.

EXERCISE	SETS	REPS	REST BETWEEN SETS
Alternate Knee Tucks (lower)	2	12–15	20 seconds
Single-Side Leg Raise (obliques)	2	12–15	20 seconds
Crunches— Knees in the Air (upper)	2	12–15	20 seconds
Back Extension (lower back)	2	12–15	20 seconds

Intermediate Abs

Once you reach this level, you may choose from any of the 25 ab exercises in the last chapter.

The routine I'm going to give you first is a sample one, featuring choices from the 15 Best Ab Exercises You Can Do Anywhere list. Feel free to replace any of the exercises with ones you prefer—but do be sure that you replace that exercise from the same category (lower, upper, obliques, lower back). You can also eliminate the lower-back exercises if you train that area on another day—it's your choice. However, do be sure to train your back.

You're going to notice that the rest period in between sets has been drastically reduced, which will make each set much more challenging. It will take some time for your body to get used to this program, so go at a relaxed pace.

SAMPLE INTERMEDIATE ROUTINE (OR LEVEL 3) #1

Frequency: 2–3 times a week

EXERCISE	SETS	REPS	REST BETWEEN SETS
Toe-Touch Crunches (lower)	3	15–20	10 seconds
Double Leg Over (obliques)	3	15–20	10 seconds
Crunches—Legs Straight Out (upper)	3	15–20	10 seconds
Back Flexion (lower back)*	3	15–20	10 seconds

*Don't train your lower back more than twice a week. If you train this area on a separate day, then make the proper adjustments to the routine.

NOW, FOR THIS NEXT ROUTINE, you're going to need access to a gym. (These exercises were chosen from the entire list of 25 in the last chapter. You can replace any of them with choices from the same category—lower, upper, oblique—but do choose from the 25 exercises listed.)

SAMPLE INTERMEDIATE ROUTINE (OR LEVEL 3) #2

Frequency: 2–3 times a week

EXERCISE	SETS	REPS	REST BETWEEN SETS
Hanging Reverse Crunch (lower)	3	15–20	10 seconds
Lying Oblique Crunch: Stability Ball (obliques)	3	15–20	10 seconds
Ball Crunch (upper)	3	15–20	10 seconds
Hyperextensions (lower back)*	3	15–20	10 seconds

*Don't train your lower back more than twice a week. If you train this area on a separate day, then make the proper adjustments to the routine.

Keep in mind that you can do these routines 3 days a week, but be sure to leave a day in between each workout. (For example, train your abs on Monday, Wednesday, and Friday.)

Advanced Abdominal Routines

The sample program below (with exercises taken from the 15 Best Ab Exercises You Can Do Anywhere list) is just one of the many different ways you can train your midsection, and you can easily change it to suit your own needs. Everyone's body responds and progresses at different rates, so it's okay to change the exercises or the order in which you do them to make it better for your body. (Note that we've added an additional exercise for the lower abs as well.)

I use the following routine for my own abs and do it four or five times a month. Why so little? Well, I constantly change my routines around to shock my abs into responding. You should do the same because your body will get used to the routine and stop responding. You need to avoid hitting a plateau.

You can replace any of the ab exercises in this chart from the same category—lower, upper, obliques—just choose from the 25 ab exercises in the last chapter. You should do this routine a minimum of 2 times a week or every other day.

SAMPLE ADVANCED ROUTINE (OR LEVEL 4) #1

Frequency: 2–4 times a week

EXERCISE	SETS	REPS	REST BETWEEN SETS
Toe-Touch Crunches (lower)	3	20–25	5 seconds
Alternate Knee Tucks (lower)	3	20–25	5 seconds
Twisting Crunch—Feet Against Wall (obliques)	3	20–25	5 seconds
Crunches: Knees in the Air (upper)	3	20–25	5 seconds
Cat and Camel (lower back)*	3	20–25	10 seconds

*Don't train your lower back more than twice a week. If you train this area on a separate day, then make the proper adjustments to the routine.

NOW, FOR THIS NEXT ROUTINE, you're going to need access to a gym. (These exercises were chosen from the entire list of 25 in the last chapter. You can replace any of the ab exercises from the same category—lower, upper, oblique—but do choose from the 25 ab exercises.) You should do this routine a minimum of 2 times a week or every other day.

SAMPLE ADVANCED ROUTINE (OR LEVEL 4) #2

Frequency: 2–4 times a week

EXERCISE	SETS	REPS	REST BETWEEN SETS
Exercise Ball Reverse Crunch (lower)	3	20	5 seconds
Bicycles (lower)	3	20	5 seconds
Hanging Twisting Leg Raises (obliques)	3	20	5 seconds
Crunch—Kneeling Rope (upper)	3	20	5 seconds
Exercise Ball—Back Extension (lower back)*	3	20	10 seconds

*Don't train your lower back more than twice a week. If you train this area on a separate day, then make the proper adjustments to the routine.

ircuit-Training Your Abs

This is a very good way to train your abs—instead of doing multiple sets for each exercise, you'll do one set of each exercise and go on to the next after your allotted rest between each set. So, for example, let's say that your first exercise is a **Basic Crunch.** If you were a beginner, you'd do 15 reps, wait 20 seconds, and then go to the next exercise. This is a simple and effective way to train abs. (Make sure that you know your routine by heart, or you'll find yourself taking too much time between each set, wondering if you should do a crunch or leg raise next.)

BEGINNER'S ROUTINE
Frequency: 2 times a week

Wait at least 48 hours between ab workouts.
All of the exercises below are from the list of 15 Ab Exercises You Can Do Anywhere.

EXERCISE	REPS	REST BETWEEN EXERCISES
1. Lying Leg Raise (lower)	12–15	20 seconds
2. Single-Side Leg Raise (obliques)	12–15	20 seconds
3. Basic Crunch (upper)	12–15	20 seconds
4. Bicycles (lower)	12–15	20 seconds
5. Cross-Knee Crunch (obliques)	12–15	20 seconds
6. Butterfly Crunch (upper)	12–15	20 seconds

Choose one back exercise and do two sets of 12–15 reps with 20 seconds of rest between sets after you finish your ab routine.

INTERMEDIATE LEVEL ROUTINE

Frequency: 2–3 times a week
(Example: Monday, Wednesday, Friday)

Leave a day between workouts for recuperation.
All of the exercises below are from the list of 15 Ab Exercises You Can Do Anywhere.*

EXERCISE	REPS	REST BETWEEN EXERCISES
1. Toe-Touch Crunches (lower)	15–20	10 seconds
2. Crunches—Legs Straight Out (upper)	15–20	10 seconds
3. Double Leg Over (obliques)	15–20	10 seconds
4. Bicycles (lower)	15–20	10 seconds
5. Basic Crunch (upper)	15–20	10 seconds
6. Twisting Crunch—Feet Against Wall (obliques)	15–20	10 seconds
7. Alternate Knee Tucks (lower)	15–20	10 seconds
8. Butterfly Crunch (upper)	15–20	10 seconds
9. Single-Side Leg Raise (obliques)	15–20	10 seconds

Choose one back exercise and do 3 sets of 20 with 10 seconds of rest between sets after you complete your abdominal routine.

*You can substitute ab exercises for the list of 15. You can also choose your exercise form the list of 25 if you have access to a gym—just make sure you pick your exercises from the right category.

SAMPLE ADVANCED LEVEL ROUTINE #1

Frequency: 2–4 times a week based on your own individual fitness level and needs.

All of the exercises below are from the list of 15 Ab Exercises You Can Do Anywhere.

EXERCISE	REPS	REST BETWEEN EXERCISES
1. Lying Leg Raise (lower)	20	5 seconds
2. Cross-Knee Crunch (obliques)	20	5 seconds
3. Basic Crunch (upper)	20	5 seconds
4. Bicycles (lower)	20	5 seconds
5. Double Leg Over (obliques)	20	5 seconds
6. Crunches—Knees in the Air (upper)	20	5 seconds
7. Toe-Touch Crunches (lower)	20	5 seconds
8. Single-Side Leg Raise (obliques)	20	5 seconds
9. Butterfly Crunch (upper)	20	5 seconds
10. Alternate Knee Tucks (lower)	20	5 seconds
11. Twisting Crunch—Feet Against Wall (obliques)	20	5 seconds
12. Crunches—Legs Straight Out (upper)	20	5 seconds

Choose one back exercise and do three sets of 20–25 reps with 10 seconds of rest between sets after you finish your ab routine.

SAMPLE ADVANCED LEVEL ROUTINE #2

Frequency: 2–4 times a week based on your own individual fitness level and needs.

If you want to follow this intermediate ab routine you are going to need access to a gym. The exercises were chosen from the list of 25.

EXERCISE	REPS	REST BETWEEN EXERCISES
1. Hanging Reverse Crunch (lower)	20	5 seconds
2. Hanging Twisting Leg Raise (obliques)	20	5 seconds
3. Exercise Ball Crunch (upper)	20	5 seconds
4. Exercise Ball Leg Lifts (lower)	20	5 seconds
5. Exercise Ball Lying Oblique Crunch (obliques)	20	5 seconds
6. Crunch—Machine (upper and lower)	20	5 seconds
7. Toe-Touch Crunches (lower)	20	5 seconds
8. Double Leg Over (obliques)	20	5 seconds
9. Kneeling Crunch—Rope (upper)	20	5 seconds
10. Exercise Ball Reverse Crunch (lower)	20	5 seconds
11. Single-Side Leg Raise (obliques)	20	5 seconds
12. Crunches—Knees in the Air (upper)	20	5 seconds

Choose one back exercise and do three sets of 20–25 reps with 10 seconds of rest between sets after you finish your ab routine.

Expert Ab Routines

If you've been training your abs for some time and aren't making any progress, then the problem might be that you're not changing your workouts frequently enough.

If you do the same routine over and over, you're wasting your time because your body gets used to the program and stops responding. There are people who do the same routine for five years—at that point, it's not about change, but maintaining what they've already got.

In my program, once you become an intermediate trainer then you really do need to switch your ab routines around during every third workout. A beginner has to learn the basics and get his or her body acclimated to the program, but once you reach intermediate level, it's time to experiment and shock your body into new development. I suggest that you add one of the techniques listed below in every third workout—they'll definitely give your abs the boost they need and stop your body from hitting a plateau.

If you're an advanced trainer, then you're probably already using these techniques in your daily workout because you know the secret: they work.

Super Sets

The first technique we're going to learn is called a *super set,* which is when you perform two different exercises consecutively without resting. Choose two different ab exercises, but don't pick two that work the same area. For example, choose one for your lower abs, and then one for your upper or obliques area. In other words, don't pick two ab exercises from the same category.

These super sets will really intensify your ab workout:

EXERCISE	REPS	REST BETWEEN SETS
Lying Leg Raises (lower)	15–20	none
Basic Crunches (upper)*	15–20	none

*After **Basic Crunches**, rest for 30 seconds, then repeat the set.

Do this super set as part of your workout; or do 3 sets of the above 2 exercises as a whole workout.

Tri-Sets

We all know that the prefix *tri* means "three," but I like to say that it means to "try hard" because these exercises will certainly take your workout up a notch!

Tri-sets are more difficult than super sets because you're performing three consecutive exercises with no rest between them. They're also great for people with limited time on their hands because they provide a very short and intense workout. (I've been known to do a tri-set of abs in my hotel room when I travel.)

When I choose abdominal exercises for my tri-set, I pick one for lower, upper, and obliques. This way, I know that I'm working the entire abdominal area and get a complete workout.

EXERCISE	REPS	REST BETWEEN SETS
Alternate Knee Tucks (lower)	**15–20**	**none**
Single Side Leg Raise (oblique)	**15–20**	**none**
Crunch—Knees in the Air (upper)*	**15–20**	**none**
*After **Crunch—Knees in the Air**, rest for 30 seconds, then repeat the set.		

This routine can constitute your entire workout (you can do between 2–4 sets depending on your current fitness level).

Giant Sets

This technique, in which you do 4 exercises in a row, is definitely not for the weak. In fact, if you thought tri-sets were hard, they're going to seem like a treat compared to what we're going to do now.

You'll pick 4 ab exercises of your choice, but make sure to include one for lower, upper, and obliques. Then you have one extra exercise to pick, which is based on your individual needs.

If your lower abs needs more work, then pick an exercise in that area. If your obliques need the extra work, then pick one that targets them. It's totally up to you.

If you do giant sets, you must give them 100 percent of your effort, but listen carefully to your body to avoid injury.

Here's one of my favorites:

EXERCISE	REPS	REST BETWEEN SETS
Hanging Reverse Crunch (lower)	15–20	none
Hanging Twisting Leg Raise (oblique)	15–20	none
Exercise Ball Crunch (upper)	15–20	none
Lying Leg Raise (lower)*	15–20	none

*After **Lying Leg Raise**, rest for 30–45 seconds, then repeat the set.

You can choose to put the exercises in any order, but I prefer to do lower abs, obliques, and then upper abs. You can mix it up until you find what works best for you.

This is a very difficult workout, and you won't have to add any additional ab work if you do it.

Ab Routines If You're Short on Time: Combining Your Abs and Weight-Training Workout

Being short on time can really affect your workout. For example, let's say that you train on your lunch break. You have one hour to train, shower, and get back to the office—obviously, you can't fit an entire workout into this time, so you find yourself rushing at the gym, which means that your quality, results, and progress suffer.

How can you get an effective ab workout when you're looking at the clock? Well, I've found that a great way to train your abs is in between the sets of your regular weight-training workout. If, for instance, you're also training your chest, then your first exercise is the **Bench Press** (which, along with other non-ab exercises, can be found in the next chapter). When you finish your set, you'll immediately perform an ab exercise. In fact, with a little planning, you can do your entire ab routine during the rest periods of your other routines.

The following routine is a perfect example of what I'm talking about:

EXAMPLE: CHEST/ABS

EXERCISE	SETS	REPS	
Bench Press	1	12	
Basic Crunch	1	20	
Bench Press	1	10	Perform the first exercise in this chart and immediately follow it with the next exercise with no rest in between. Rest 30 seconds, then move on to the next group of two exercises, and so on, with 30-second breaks in between each group.
Basic Crunch	1	20	
Bench Press	1	8	
Basic Crunch	1	20	
Incline Fly	1	12	
Lying Leg Raise	1	20	
Incline Fly	1	10	
Lying Leg Raise	1	20	
Incline Fly	1	8	
Lying Leg Raise	1	20	

This is just one way you can do this routine. If you're following an ab-circuit routine, then you'll be doing a different ab exercise after each of your strength-training exercises. If you're not following a circuit and are following a basic ab routine, then do your routine as written between the strength exercises. If you're really short on time, you can use the super-set method. I wouldn't recommend doing a tri-set or giant set because it will take too long to perform and will take away significantly from your strength and stamina. It will also hurt your weight-training workout.

Strength-Training Your Abs by Adding Resistance

This section won't apply to everyone, as most of you will build enough ab strength through the routines we've already discussed in the book. As far as achieving a six-pack goes, we know that an ab workout is only part of the equation: You also need to diet, do cardio, and perform other exercises.

This portion is important to athletes of all sports and people who want to improve their posture. I do believe that at some point everyone should be adding some resistance to their ab workouts, especially those who have reached the advanced level.

So here we'll be focusing on building additional abdominal strength. Training your abs with resistance has many benefits, including strengthening and stimulating the growth of your muscles. I've already told you that when it comes to abs, more isn't necessarily better. Many people are under the impression that if they can do 100 crunches easily, then they must have strong abs. They might have stronger and better conditioned muscles than when they started, but it's time to move on. If you can easily do 100 reps of *any* exercise, you're not using enough resistance to increase your muscle strength.

When everyone starts out, their individual body weight is enough to fatigue the ab muscles with 15 or 20 reps. Once you accomplish those 15–20 reps, it's time to increase your overload (by adding weight) so that you can fatigue your abs without having to do 700 reps. You still want to stay between 12 and 20 reps, which will keep you in *stimulation range,* rather than *conditioning range.* You also don't want to go too heavy, so I advise you to avoid low-rep sets, since you can get injured very easily.

Here are 3 tips to help with this:

Tips on Adding Resistance to Your Ab Exercises

1.   Hold weight plates in front of or behind your body.
2.   Use resistance bands.
3.   Use ab machines with added weight stacks.

Couples Training

I've found that having a partner can be very beneficial for training. When there's a physical attraction between you and that person, it's even better.

Now I'm not saying that you should run out and find a girl- or boyfriend in order to train abs. But if you've got a little crush on the person on the other side of you, it will make training fun. He or she should also make sure your form is correct, keep you in rhythm, make sure your breathing is correct, and count your reps.

I love training abs with my wife, Lisa. Not only do I get the ab benefits, but it's also a form of sexual foreplay because of the closeness and touching going on throughout. It also makes the session go very quickly. (I'm smiling right now just thinking about it.) But with any partner, I concentrate more and train more intensely. Maybe it's the competitive thing, or it's about someone looking over at you that makes you more consciously aware of what you're doing—whatever it is, I highly recommend that you try it.

What I Do

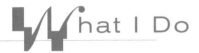

Although I change up my own routine quite frequently, what follows is what I do most of the time (please note that I do super sets of some exercises):

MY AB ROUTINE

EXERCISE	SETS	REPS	REST BETWEEN SETS
Exercise Ball Reverse Crunch (lower)	3	20	**5 seconds**
Hanging Twisting Leg Raises (obliques)	3	20	**5 seconds**
SUPER SETS OF THE FOLLOWING:*			
Exercise Ball Crunch (upper)	1	20	**20 seconds**
Lying Leg Raise (lower)	1	20	**between sets**
Exercise Ball Back Extension (lower back)	3	20	**10 seconds**

*I do 3 super sets each.

I ALSO SPEND A LOT OF TIME on the road, but that doesn't mean that I have to let my abs slip. Whether or not I can make it to the gym doesn't affect my workout—as long as I have enough room on the floor, I'm ready to go.

It's safe to say that when I'm traveling my time is limited, so my objective is a great, effective ab workout in as short a time as possible. I find that super sets are the way to go:

MY HOTEL-ROOM WORKOUT

EXERCISE	SETS	REPS	REST BETWEEN SETS
SUPER SET 1*			
Lying Leg Raises (lower)	1	20	**20 seconds**
Crunches—Knees in the Air (upper)	1	20	**between sets**
SUPER SET 2*			
Alternate Knee Tucks (lower)	1	20	**20 seconds**
Twisting Crunch—Feet Against Wall (obliques)	1	20	**between sets**
Back Flexion (lower back)	3	20	**20 seconds between sets**

*I do 3 super sets each.

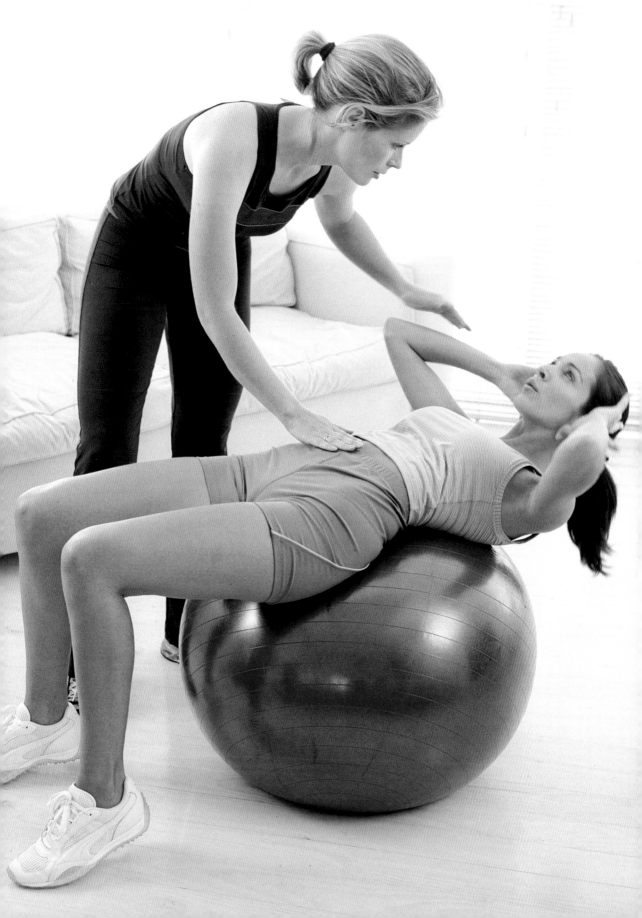

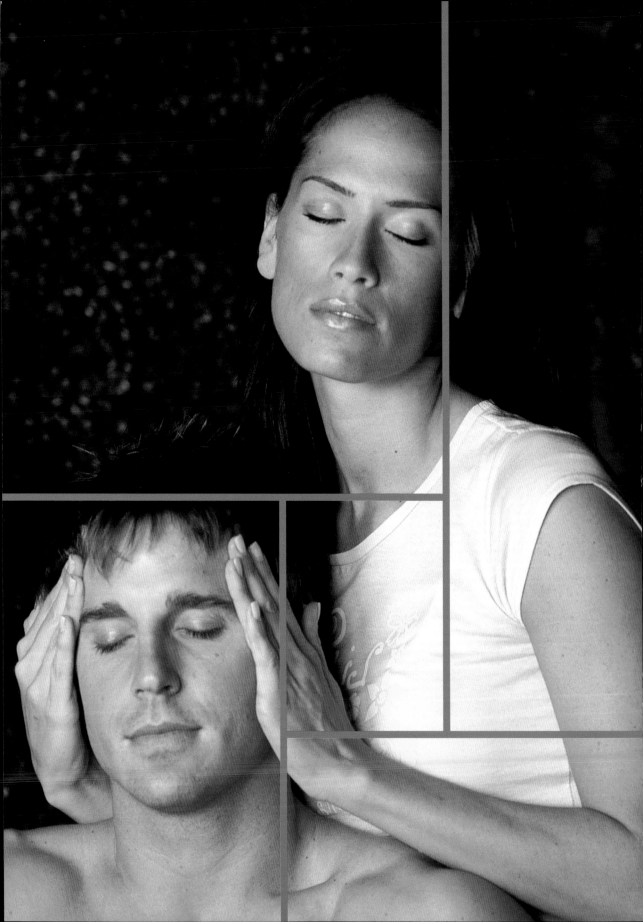

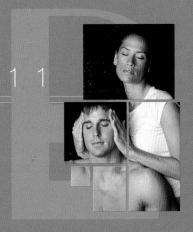

CHAPTER 11

BEYOND ABS

We've come a long way, but we're not finished yet!

Let's go back to the idea of intentions: My intention for you isn't just to build a great set of abs—I also want you to embrace a healthier lifestyle. After all, the primary goal of any exercise program should be to maintain or improve your health.

If you follow the nutrition and cardio hints while doing the abdominal routines contained in this book, you'll become healthier and your abs will become toned. But what about the rest of you? A shapely body and a toned midsection go together. I mean, you don't want to look like you're wearing one of those fake-ab T-shirts, right? Well, I'm sorry to report that you won't get a great physique from just doing ab exercises—you need to add a weight/resistance-training workout to your program, too. Working out with weights will dramatically improve the look of your body, while resistance training will help you develop more self-confidence and body contentment.

In other words, you'll be building and toning those once-flabby muscles, and at the same time, you'll increase your strength and endurance. Resistance training also decreases your risk of osteoporosis, helps you prevent injury, and ensures that you maintain lean body mass. Each of those components are important for people who are trying to lose weight.

Now, let's figure out a few ways to get your entire body in shape.

What about Yoga and Pilates?

I generally don't frown upon any activity that gets a person off the couch and moving. But having said that, I definitely believe that some exercise routines are better then others.

Let's start with yoga, especially Bikram yoga, which is done in a room with the temperature hovering around 120 degrees. I attend twice-weekly classes, as I find the practice a great way to improve flexibility, strengthen muscles, and clear my mind. However, yoga isn't as effective for building and sculpting muscles as weight training is.

Yoga will give you a more limber and flexible body, which will increase your circulation, help prevent injuries, and make daily activities easier to do. It will also improve your posture, give you added definition, and help improve your mental state. But when you're performing yoga, you're working with your own body's weight. In other words, you can get a good workout, but you'll be limited because it's the overload of weight that builds and strengthens muscles. Weight training, on the other hand, allows you to constantly challenge and shock your body because there's no limit to how much weight you can use. It will also help you build lean mass, change the symmetry of your body for the better, and give you more muscular endurance and strength.

I find that the perfect routine includes both weights and yoga, but if you have to choose only one, I'd go for the weight training.

THERE ARE TWO TYPES OF PILATES: machine-based and mat programs. Machine-based Pilates is similar to weight training because it involves moving against resistance with the goal of overloading the muscles; while the mat class is similar to yoga because you use your own body for resistance. Yet Pilates is better than yoga if you want to change the look of your body. (I'd choose the machine class over the mat one to build strength and muscle.)

I've attended a few Pilates classes and thought it was funny that the instructor kept blasting weight training. I was told that using weights shortens muscles, while Pilates lengthens them—that's just not true, as *all* muscles lengthen in a relaxed state. I also heard that Pilates corrects muscular imbalances, heals back injuries, and will help you realign your body, while weight training won't do any of that. Well, that's not true either: If weight training is performed correctly, it will do all of the above.

Even though Pilates will help you get in shape, it comes down to personal preferences: I prefer weight training because I know all the positive things it has done for me and millions of other people; plus, I've never seen or heard of any Olympic or professional athlete who has excluded some form of weight training from his or her program.

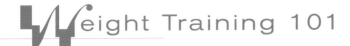eight Training 101

Okay, now that you've made the commitment to start a weight-training program and are ready to transform that once-flabby body into a toned and sleek physique, the first thing you're going to have to decide is where you're going to train: at home or at the gym.

Let's examine the pros and cons of each choice in further detail.

Training at Home

There are many people who think that you have to join an expensive gym or get a top personal trainer in order to succeed at being fit. I trained in my basement for four years before I even went to a commercial gym, and I made some fantastic strides there. Especially if you're just starting out, you can get a fantastic workout by training at home. It also makes perfect sense: You might be one of those people who has no time to get to a gym because of work, the kids, or your mate, so why not bring the gym to you?

If you make the decision to train at home, you're going to have to purchase some equipment, so make sure that you're serious about getting in shape before you make the investment. (Remember the joke I told earlier about having the world's most expensive coatrack.)

There are hundreds of home-gym systems out there, but I'd start with buying some basic dumb- and barbells, which won't break the bank. If you can afford a total-body-workout system, then I suggest that you try it out before you buy it—after all, you don't want to spend $1,000 and be disappointed. I do believe that some of these systems are good and effective, but the cheapest way you can tone your body is with free weights. Believe me, they work.

The following workout can easily be done at home. All you need are the following items:

1. A flat bench—price estimate: $100*
2. A pair of adjustable dumbbells—price estimate: from $40–$90
(*Of course, prices vary. Check out your newspaper's classified section because gyms are always upgrading equipment and people constantly sell fitness equipment they never use. For less than $200, you can train at home and have a great workout.)

I also hope that training at home will motivate you to join a gym and inspire you to explore other workout routines and options. But even if you do, it's helpful to keep those weights around the house. I use mine in bad weather or if I get home too late to hit the gym. It's better than sitting around watching TV.

Training in a Gym

Now, if you decide to train in a gym, choosing the right one is very important. After all, if you're not in an environment that's positive and you don't enjoy being there, then it's going to have a negative impact on your progress.

You can definitely purchase an affordable membership, but don't tie yourself into a long deal because things change. You might switch jobs and find a new gym closer to you, or you might not like some of the members. It happens. My advice is to join for a few months; then, if you like it, you can sign up for a yearly membership. Most gyms let you re-up for no additional cost.

So what should you look for when choosing a gym? The following list should help:

1. **Location, location, location.** Make sure that the gym you're considering fits geographically into your lifestyle; in other words, it should be close to your home or job. If it's far away, you either won't go or you'll go far less frequently.

2. **Variety.** Choose a gym with weight training, aerobic classes, yoga, and a huge selection of cardio equipment—you'll want as many fitness options as possible to stave off boredom.

3. **Cleanliness.** Pick a gym that has immaculate bathrooms and equipment. I mean, the point of going to a gym is to get healthier—not to pick up a fungus or virus from the facility.

4. **Price.** There are so many gyms around today that they're all fighting for members. But don't let a fast-talking salesman force you into a package—take your time and shop around. There are usually deals for every season, so enjoy any trial-week memberships you can find. Go every single day to experience how the particular gym changes, remember if you have to wait to use the equipment, and check out the other members.

5. **Parking.** The last thing you want to do is drive around for 20 minutes looking for a spot. Make sure that your gym has enough parking, even during peak hours.

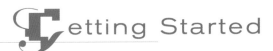 # Getting Started

Now that you've chosen your place of exercise, it's time to get started. Keep in mind that the very first thing you should do is warm up—most people get hurt because they fail to properly and thoroughly do so before starting a weight program. The simple fact is that cold muscles tear, so please warm up before you train. If you don't think you have the time, I'll bet that you also don't have the time for an injury.

Here's what I suggest:

Daily Warm-up

1. First, do **5 minutes of the cardio exercise** of your choice. This is a warm-up, not the Boston marathon, so take it easy.

2. Next, do a **full-body stretching routine for 5 minutes.** Stretching has numerous benefits, such as helping to reduce the physical stress you'll be putting on your muscles. Make sure that you stretch your whole body: Hold each stretch for 5–10 seconds; move slowly and don't bounce; and stretch until the muscle feels tight. Never stretch until you feel pain.

A Few Questions about Lifting

As a personal trainer, I've found that there are three very popular questions I'm asked whenever someone comes to the gym for the first time. (You veterans out there should also read this in case someone asks you the same questions.) Here they are:

Question #1: "How do I pick the right weight to lift?"
Frank says: The only way you're going to figure out how much weight you should use for any particular exercise is by trial and error—that means actually lifting a weight and doing a set. Start out by picking up the lightest weight and move on from there: If you start curling and find that you can do 100 reps, then it's obviously too light. Know that it takes time to find the right weight.

Question #2: "How do I know when to increase the weight?"
Frank says: If your workout program indicates that you're supposed to do 10 reps and you get to that number easily, then it's a eureka moment: It's time to add weight. If a weight becomes too easy for you, you're not building strength or causing enough overload to build muscle. This isn't rocket science: Don't let that trainer in the gym convince you that this is a difficult process.

Question #3: "How long should I rest between sets?"
Frank says: This is based on your fitness level, but I strongly suggest that if you're just starting out, it helps to rest for 90 seconds between sets or until your normal breathing pattern returns.

Time to Train

Okay—now that that's out of the way, let's work out by following the very basic exercise program listed here.

In my first book, *The TRUTH,* I explained five levels of training and a way to develop your own personalized program for your individual body type. Of course, I can't do that here or this book would be about 1,000 pages long. But don't despair, my friends: I will give you a full-body workout here, consisting of 10 exercises that you can do at home or at the gym with a bench and some dumbbells. This routine will help you create a stronger, symmetrical, more toned physique, and it will speed up the development of that six-pack you've always wanted. You can't beat that, right?

28 DAY-WORKOUT PLAN: AT HOME OR THE GYM

PROGRAM DURATION: **28 days**

WORKOUT FREQUENCY:
3 days a week

WORKOUT TYPE: **Full body**

EXERCISES PER DAY: **10**

SETS OF EACH EXERCISE:
2 (beginners), 3–4 for more advanced people

REPETITION SCHEME: **12–15 reps per set (beginners); 10–12 reps (intermediate-advanced)**

REST BETWEEN SETS: **90 seconds (beginners); 60 seconds (intermediate/ advanced)**

PERFORM AS A CIRCUIT: **No rest in between sets (advanced)**

DAILY WARM-UP:
Cardio
5 minutes at low intensity
Stretching
Full-body stretch for 5 minutes

SAMPLE PROGRAM (BEGINNERS)

EXERCISE	SETS	REPS	REST BETWEEN SETS
Bench Press (chest)	2	12–15	90 seconds
Fly (chest)	2	12–15	90 seconds
One-Arm Row (back)	2	12–15	90 seconds
Shoulder Press (shoulders)	2	12–15	90 seconds
Side Raise (shoulders)	2	12–15	90 seconds
Biceps Curl (biceps)	2	12–15	90 seconds
Overhead Triceps Extension (triceps)	2	12–15	90 seconds
Squat (legs)	2	12–15	90 seconds
Stiff-Legged Dead Lift (lower back, hamstrings)	2	12–15	90 seconds
Standing Calf Raise (calves)	2	12–15	90 seconds

Notes: After you complete all 10 exercises, go back and start from #1 and do another set for each (complete 2 sets for each exercise). Do your ab routine after this workout—go to the ab-routine section in Chapter 10 to pick out your exercises. And don't forget your cardio!

Detailed descriptions of the exercises listed above begin on page 161, along with photos that will help you ensure that you're using proper form.

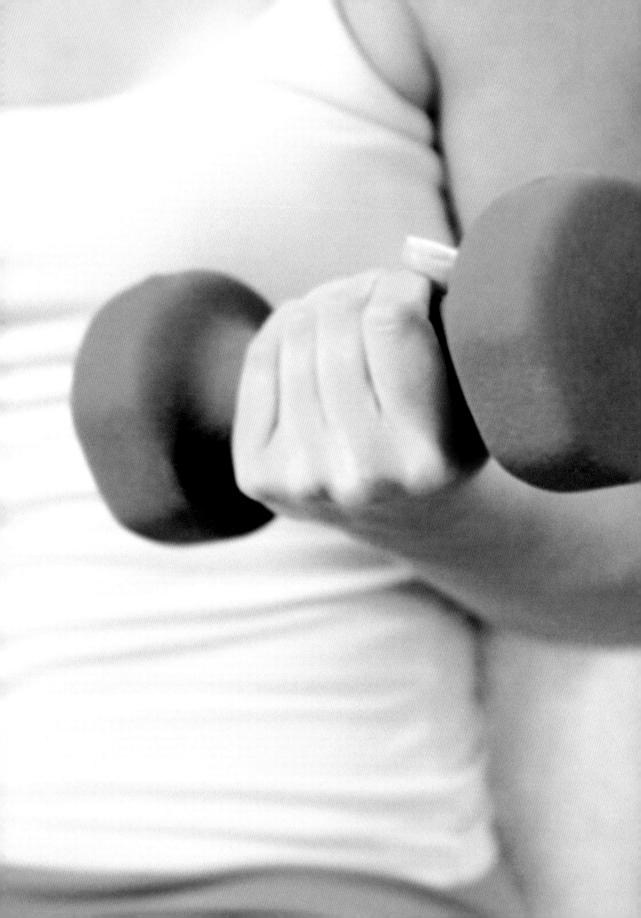

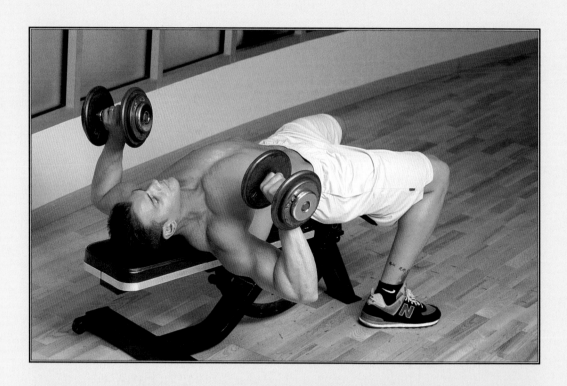

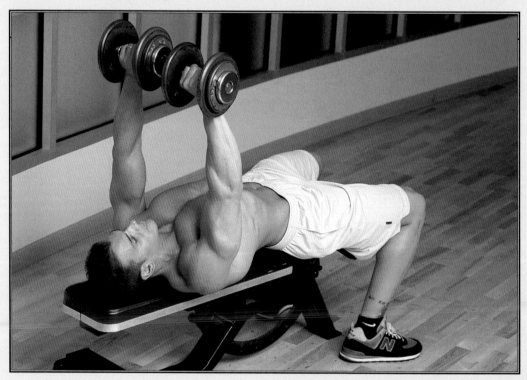

Bench Press

Sit on the end of a flat bench with your feet flat on the floor. Hold a dumbbell upright in each hand, with the weight of the dumbbell resting on your upper thighs. Lie back on the bench and tilt the dumbbells back off your thighs so that their weight is transferred to your hands. With the dumbbells held just above your chest, turn your wrists, so that instead of facing each other, your palms face toward your feet. Inhale as you slowly press the dumbbells upward and slightly toward each other until your arms are fully extended (but your elbows aren't locked). Exhale as you slowly lower the dumbbells back to just above your chest.

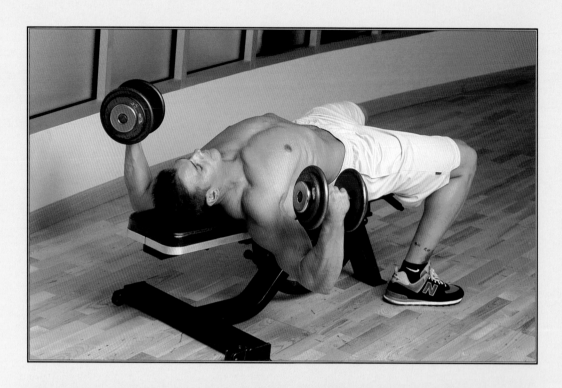
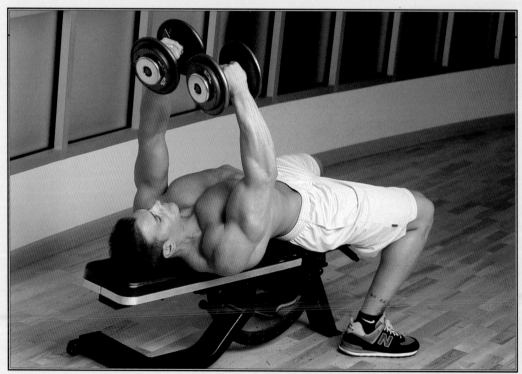

Fly

Sit on the end of a flat bench with feet flat on the floor. Hold a dumbbell upright in each hand, with the weight of the dumbbells resting on your upper thighs. Lie back on the bench as you lift the dumbbells off your thighs. Press them up until they're at arm's length directly over your chest, with your elbows bent at a 10-degree angle. Turn the dumbbells so that your palms are facing each other. Maintaining the bend in your elbows, inhale as you slowly lower the dumbbells straight out to your sides, as low as you can go. Exhale as you slowly lift the dumbbells back up high over your chest.

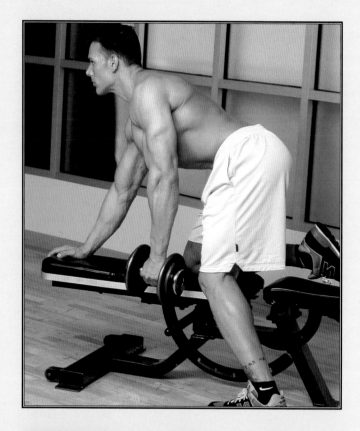

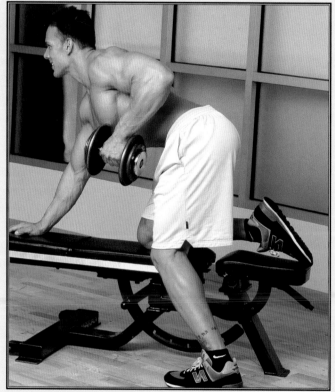

One-Arm Row

Stand on the left side of a bench with a dumbbell on the floor in front of you. Rest your right knee and shin on the bench. Bend forward and plant your right hand on the bench, so that your back is parallel to the floor. Grasp the dumbbell with your left hand, palm facing your body. Inhale as you slowly lift the dumbbell up to your side. Exhale as you slowly lower the dumbbell to just above the floor. Finish your reps, move to the right side of the bench, and repeat the exercise with your right arm.

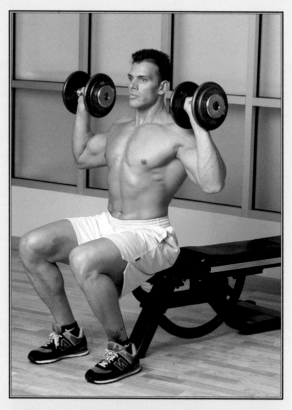

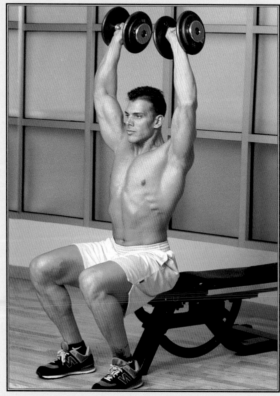

Shoulder Press

Sit with your feet flat on the floor and a dumbbell in each hand, resting upright on your thighs. Lift the dumbbells up to just above your shoulders, rotating them so that they're parallel to the floor, your palms facing forward and your elbows directly below your wrists. Inhale as you slowly press the barbells up until your arms are fully extended (but elbows aren't locked). Then exhale as you slowly lower the dumbbells back to just above your shoulders.

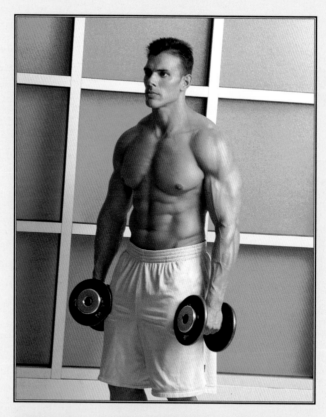

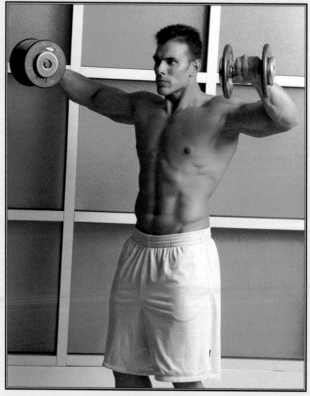

Side Raise

Hold two dumbbells next to your thighs with your arms fully extended. Have a slight bend in your elbows and your palms facing each other. Standing with your knees slightly bent and your feet shoulder-width apart, bend very slightly forward at the hips. Inhale as you slowly lift both dumbbells directly out to your sides until your elbows are at shoulder height. Your palms should be facing down. Exhale as you slowly lower the dumbbells back to your sides.

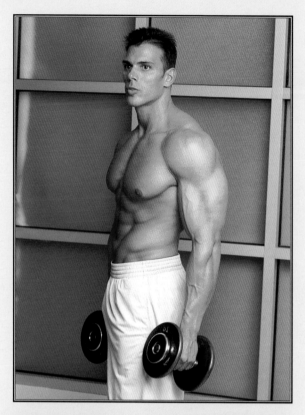

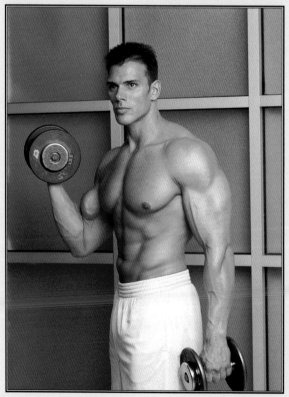

Biceps Curl

Stand with your feet shoulder-width apart and knees slightly bent. Hold a dumbbell in each hand, palms facing each other. With your elbows pointing straight down and held in tight to your sides, inhale and lift your right forearm, slowly curling the dumbbell up toward your chest until your biceps are fully contracted. As you curl the dumbbell up, rotate it so that your palm is facing up at the top of the motion. Exhale as you slowly lower the dumbbell back to your side, rotating it back so that your palm faces your side. Repeat the motion with your left arm.

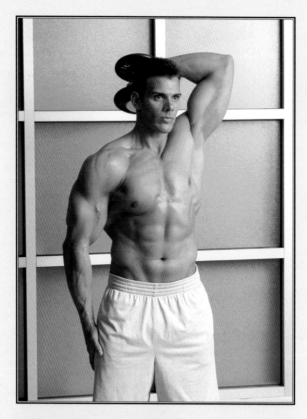

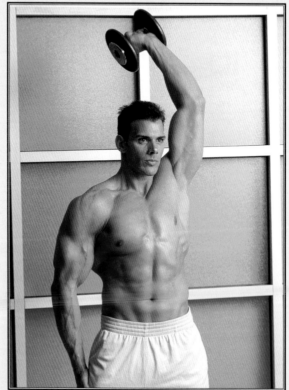

Overhead Triceps Extension

Stand with feet shoulder-width apart and knees slightly bent, with a dumbbell in your left hand and your right arm at your side. Raise the dumbbell so that your left arm is extended straight up. Keeping your upper arm pointed straight up, inhale as you slowly lower the dumbbell back behind your head. Then exhale as you lift the dumbbell back up until your arm is fully extended, your elbow locked. Complete your reps, switch arms, and perform the exercise with your right arm.

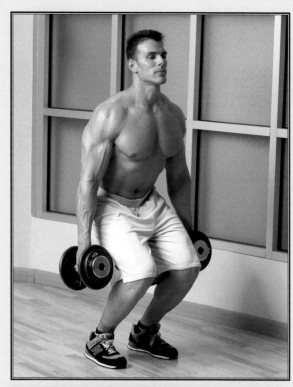

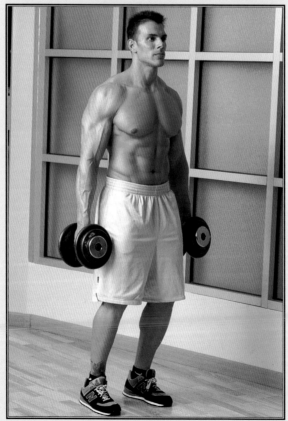

Squat

Stand with your feet shoulder-width apart, with your toes and knees slightly pointing out-ward. Hold dumbbells in your hands with your arms at your sides. Keeping your back straight and your head up, squat down until your thighs are parallel to the floor. Inhale as you bend at the knees and hips, slowly lowering your butt back and behind you until your thighs are paral-lel to the floor. Exhale as you slowly press back up to the starting position.

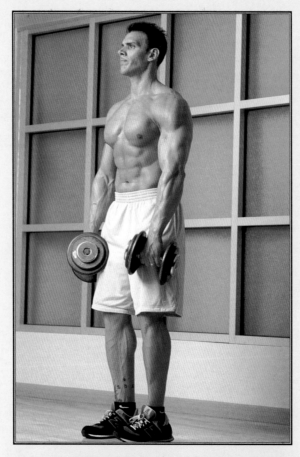
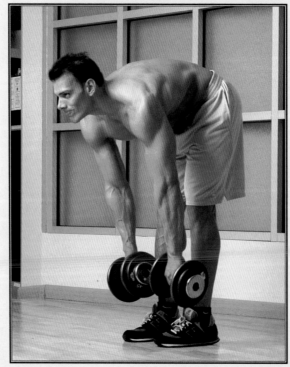

Stiff-Legged Dead Lift

Hold a dumbbell in each hand with an overhand grip, hands shoulder-width apart. Stand with your feet shoulder-width apart and your knees locked, the dumbbells resting against your thighs, and your arms fully extended. With your back straight, bend forward from the waist to the starting position, with your upper body parallel to the floor. The dumbbells should be hanging at arm's length below your shoulders. Keeping your knees locked, inhale as you slowly lift your torso and stand up straight, the dumbbells hanging in front of your upper thighs. Exhale as you slowly bend forward and lower your torso back to parallel with the floor.

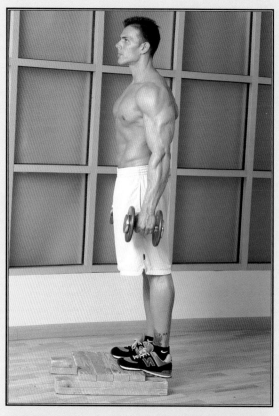

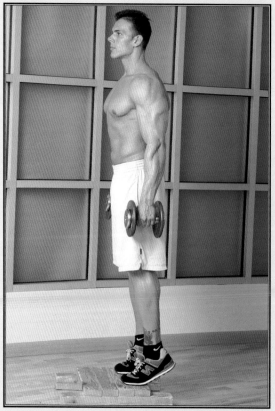

Standing Calf Raise

Place a wooden block (or something similar that's two to three inches tall) on the ground. Grasp a dumbbell in each hand. Position your toes and the balls of your feet on the block, with arches and heels extending off and resting on the floor. Raise your heels by extending your ankles as high as possible, then lower your heels by bending your ankles until your calves are stretched. Inhale as you press up from your toes, slowly lifting your heels as high as you can above the level of the wooden block. Exhale as you slowly lower your heels as far down below the wooden block as you can.

IN THE NAME OF PROGRESS, this general full-body workout can be made much more difficult just by using heavier weights and cutting down on your rest intervals between sets. But don't do so right away, as it will take some time for your body to get adjusted to the program. I believe that you should make the program harder when you complete 12 workouts within 28 days.

For those of you who are more advanced and are looking for a more difficult workout, add some sets or heavier reps like I suggested above. You can also do this in circuit form with no rest in between sets. Believe me when I tell you that's a very challenging workout.

Hopefully, you'll reach a point where you want more out of your weight-training session— that's when we'll add exercises and sets while training each body part on a particular day. I believe that when your reach that point, you'll have made some wonderful progress and built a great foundation by using the 10-exercise program I've given you.

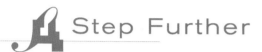 Step Further

For those of you who are ready to tackle the next phase of training, I've provided you with a sample of a gym-only workout from my book *The TRUTH*. If you want to learn everything about how to individualize your workout specifically for your body type and fitness level, then you should definitely pick up a copy.

SAMPLE INTERMEDIATE (OR LEVEL 3) PROGRAM

PROGRAM DURATION: 28 days

WORKOUT FREQUENCY:
  4 days a week

WORKOUT TYPE: Full body

DAILY WARM-UP:
Cardio
  5 minutes low intensity
Stretching
  Full-body stretch for 5 minutes

Level 3: Sample Week

DAY 1

BACK (9 sets)
Bent-Over Row—Barbell
3 sets of 12, 10, and 8 reps
**Row—Cable with
V-Handle**
3 sets of 12, 10, and 8 reps
Lat Pull-Down—Front
3 sets of 12, 10, and 8 reps

ABS (6 sets)
**Refer to Chapter 10 of
this book for appropriate
exercises**

DAY 2

SHOULDERS (9 sets)
**Front Military Press—
Barbell**
3 sets of 12, 10, and 8 reps
**Shoulder Press—
Dumbbell**
3 sets of 12, 10, and 8 reps
Side Raise—Dumbbell
3 sets of 15, 12, and 10 reps

TRICEPS (6 sets)
Narrow-Grip Bench Press
3 sets of 12, 10, and 8 reps
Kickback—Dumbbell
3 sets of 15, 12, and 10 reps

ABS (6 sets)
**Refer to Chapter 10 of this
book for appropriate exercises**

DAY 3

OFF

DAY 4

UPPER LEGS (9 sets)
Squat—Machine
3 sets of 12, 10, and 8 reps
Leg Press—Machine
3 sets of 12, 10, and 8 reps
**Prone Hamstring Curl—
Dumbbell**
3 sets of 15, 12, and 10 reps

CALVES (6 sets)
**Standing Calf Raise—
Machine**
3 sets of 12, 10, and 8 reps
**Seated Calf Raise—
Machine**
3 sets of 15, 12, and 10 reps

DAY 5

CHEST (9 sets)
Bench Press—Barbell
3 sets of 12, 10, and 8 reps
Incline Press—Barbell
3 sets of 12, 10, and 8 reps
Fly—Pec Deck
3 sets of 15, 12, and 10 reps

BICEPS (6 sets)
Biceps Curl—Barbell
3 sets of 12, 10, and 8 reps
**Concentration Curl—
Dumbbell**
3 sets of 15, 12, and 10 reps

ABS (6 sets)
**Refer to Chapter 10 of this
book for appropriate
exercises**

DAY 6

OFF

DAY 7

OFF

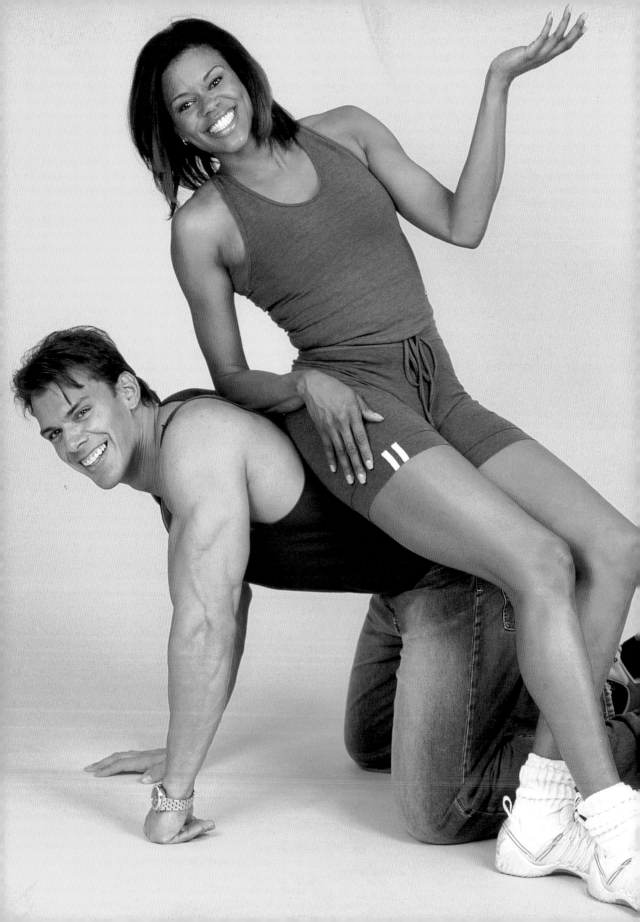

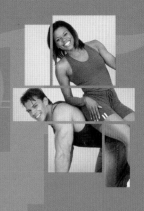

CHAPTER 12

FRANK'S FRIENDS

Let's face it: We're all human, and we each have certain things that we can't help doing. For me, it's knowing the business of my friends and neighbors.

I'm a busybody—I admit it. I ask about restaurants, clothing, what's going on with wives and husbands . . . I think it's only natural to ask someone who looks fantastic what they do to stay that way. The truth is that no one knows everything about a certain subject, so we should all be open to hearing others' opinions or ideas. So I thought that instead of giving you a boring old Afterword from me, it would be a cool idea to end this book by giving you a look at what some of my friends are doing to keep their own great abs.

The following people aren't in this book to endorse my routines or to tell you that their regimen is the greatest—they just wanted to share information on what they're doing to achieve a better midsection. (Please note that many of the exercises listed here aren't contained in either this book or *The TRUTH,* so if you're interested in doing them, you can e-mail me at **mail@franksepe.com** or **fjsepe@aol.com** for further information.)

Check out what my friends have to say, and try a few of their routines. If you come up with a great plan of your own, feel free to drop me a line. God bless, and here's to a sensational six-pack.

[**Editor's note:** All stories have been edited for space and clarity.]

John Edward

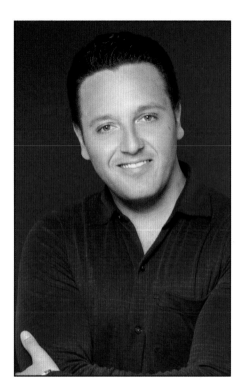

John Edward is an internationally acclaimed psychic medium and author of the *New York Times* bestsellers *One Last Time, Crossing Over, After Life, What If God Were the Sun?*, and *Final Beginnings* (with Natasha Stoynoff). In addition to hosting his own syndicated television show, *Crossing Over with John Edward,* John has been a frequent guest on *Larry King Live* and countless other talk shows. He was also featured in the HBO documentary *Life after Life.*

"I recently lost 20 pounds training with Frank Sepe, and my basic plan is to follow the ab routine he wants to torture me with that day," John says with a laugh.

JOHN EDWARD'S FAVORITE AB ROUTINE

Frequency: 2–3 times a week

EXERCISE	SETS	REPS	REST BETWEEN SETS
Bicycles (lower)	3	15–20	10 seconds
Double Leg Over (obliques)	3	15–20	10 seconds
Crunches—Legs Straight Out (upper)	3	15–20	10 seconds
Back Flexion (Lower Back)	3	15–20	10 seconds

Mike Ruiz

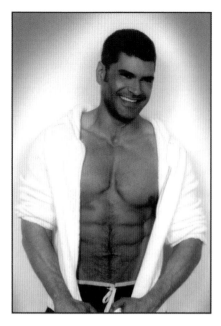

New York–based photographer Mike Ruiz was named as one of the 50 most beautiful people by *People en Español*. Mike is best known for his high-impact, colorful celebrity photography as well as his fashion editorials. He frequently shoots the hottest new stars for major American and foreign magazines including *Vanity Fair, Flaunt, Cream, Ocean Drive, Movieline's Hollywood Life, CondeNast Traveler, Interview, Latina Paper, The Source, TV Guide, XXL, V-Life,* and *Wired.* Mike has also shot advertising campaigns for Bongo jeans, MAC cosmetics, and Candies shoes. He works with music giants Arista, RCA, Interscope, TommyBoy Records, EMI, Universal, Sony, and Warner Brothers Records; along with the UPN, USA, and Sci-Fi television networks. And he's recently branched out as a director, creating music videos for Traci Lords and Kristine W. The list of celebrities that Mike has worked with reads like a Who's Who of the entertainment industry, including Jennifer Lopez, Britney Spears, Kirsten Dunst, Tyra Banks, Vin Diesel, Daryl Hannah, and Mark Wahlberg, to name a few.

"It's important to me to stay in great shape year-round. I constantly change my ab routine, and here's what I'm doing now," Mike shares.

MIKE RUIZ'S FAVORITE AB ROUTINE
Frequency: 3–4 times a week

EXERCISE	SETS
Crunch—Decline Bench	2 sets to failure (short rest in between sets)
Cable Crunch	2 sets to failure (short rest in between sets)
Exercise Ball Crunch	2 sets to failure (short rest in between sets)
Exercise Ball Leg Lifts	2 sets to failure (short rest in between sets)

Jason Fabini

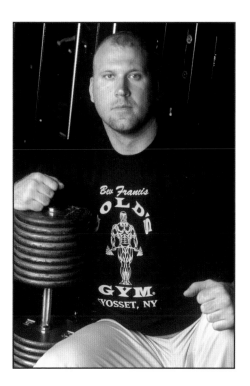

If you're a New York football fan, then you probably know Jason Fabini—for everyone else, he's an offensive tackle for the New York Jets. He's started every game he's played since 1998, which isn't an easy feat in the NFL. Besides being one of the top left tackles in the game, Jason hosts a football camp with NFL Pro Bowler Rod Woodson in Ft. Wayne, Indiana. The camp is dedicated to giving young players a chance to learn all the aspects of the game, from the weight room to the playing field.

Jason says, "Being an offensive lineman in the NFL, my main concern isn't to have a six-pack—it's keeping my core strong for the season so that my midsection can take all the hits."

JASON FABINI'S FAVORITE AB ROUTINE

EXERCISE	SETS	REPS
Medicine Ball Twist	3	15–20
Abdominal Crunch Machine (weighted)	3	15–20
Jackknives	3	15–20

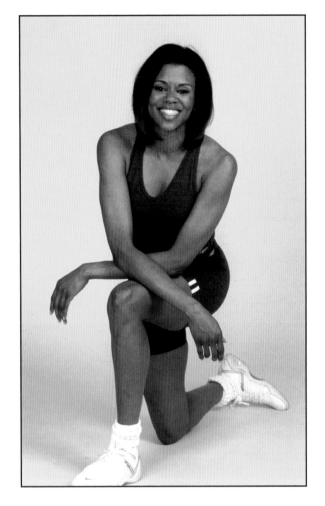

Leslie Maxie

In her first year as a reporter, Leslie was the host and anchor for Fox Sports Network and covered stories for CBS during the NCAA men's basketball championship. She's also served as anchor on the *Best Damn Sports Show Period* and has covered the Super Bowl, the NCAA's Final Four, the World Series, the NBA's All-Star Game, college football, the Rose Bowl, and baseball for The National Sports Report. In addition, she had the honor of conducting the last interview the great Jesse Owens gave to the media, and was also chosen to cover the 1988 Olympics in Seoul, South Korea.

Leslie attended the University of Southern California, where she studied public administration and received the Outstanding Student Athlete award. Currently one of the hosts of ESPN2's morning show *Cold Pizza,* she also has two children, Andrea and Nicholas. "My routine is aimed at keeping my core area strong. Since I have scoliosis in my back, the stronger it stays, the less it will curve as I grow older." Leslie adds, "I have two very active children, so I need to keep up with them because my hours are so hectic. Besides doing the routines from Frank's books, I love to use workout tapes at home to achieve my goals. Not to nag him, but I'm waiting for Frank to film one. Hurry up!" (*Note from Frank:* Leslie didn't give me any specific routine to follow.)

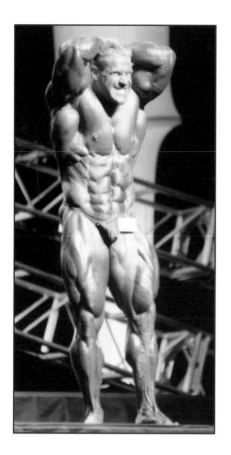

Jay Cutler

Jay is an amazing athlete and one of the best bodybuilders in the entire world. He competes at a weight of 265 pounds, and has 22½-inch arms and an astonishingly small 34-inch waist. Jay has won the prestigious Arnold Schwarzenegger Classic Bodybuilding Show an amazing three times; he's also won the Ironman Invitational, Night of Champions, and numerous Grand Prix events. In addition, he's one of the most in-demand bodybuilders for seminars and guest posings.

"I do the following routine only twice a week, and it keeps me in top shape," he says.

JAY CUTLER'S FAVORITE AB ROUTINE

Frequency: 2 times a week

EXERCISE	SETS	REPS	REST BETWEEN SETS
Hanging Twisting Leg Raise	3	15	short rest
Kneeling Crunch—Rope	3	15	between
Bench Crunches	3	15	sets

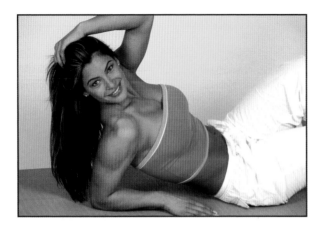

Davana Medina

Davana is one of the most sought-after fitness models in the industry. She's appeared in dozens of magazines, as well as on the cover of *Oxygen* and *MuscleMag International.* Davana competes in the International Federation of BodyBuilders (IFBB) figure contests, where competitors are judged in a bikini on their shape, conditioning, and overall look. She has the look that not only pleases her fans but the judges as well, since she's placed first in the 2003 IFBB Figure Olympia, making her the number one figure competitor in the world. She's also placed first in the 2003 Night of Champions, first in the 2003 New York Pro Show, first in the 2001 Bev Francis Atlantic State, and is the first ever figure national champion. This is one competitor who's on a winning streak that won't end anytime soon.

"When it comes to abs, I do a lot of different routines," Davana says. "I hate doing the same one over and over because, as we all know, it's boring. I do like to train abs in the fastest way possible, which is why I love Frank's program. I'm fond of doing giant sets, which means that I do 4 ab exercises in a row with no rest. It's not as bad as it sounds!"

DAVANA MEDINA'S FAVORITE AB ROUTINE (GIANT SETS)

EXERCISE	SETS	REPS
Reverse Crunch	1	20
Hanging Twisting Leg Raises	1	20
Exercise Ball Crunch	1	20
Lying Leg Raises (Exercise Ball)	1	20

Derek Panza

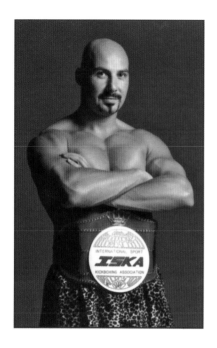

Derek is a three-time World Kickboxing Champion and is undefeated as a professional boxer. He owns and runs Panza Kickboxing Studio NY, a unique martial arts experience. Specializing in boxing, kickboxing, and submission fighting, Panza Kickboxing is set in the practical and effective training environment of a classic boxing gym and organized in the tradition of a classic martial arts school.

"Because kickboxing is a full-body sport and requires strong abs as well as strong hip flexors, my routine doesn't isolate abs," Derrick says. "I prefer to utilize abdominal muscles along with hip flexors—this helps strengthen the muscles used when kicking, which is my goal. I do the following four times a week."

DEREK PANZA'S FAVORITE AB ROUTINE

MONDAY	TUESDAY	WEDS.	THURSDAY	FRIDAY
Jackknives 50 reps **Crunches—Feet Off Floor** 50 reps **REST ONE MINUTE** **Jackknives** 25 reps **Crunches—Feet Off Floor** 50 reps **REST ONE MINUTE** **Sideways Hyperextensions (Obliques)** 2 sets, each side to failure	**3 SUPER SETS:** **Sit-Ups on a Vertical Decline** 25 reps **Hanging Leg Raises** To failure	**OFF**	**Jackknives** 50 reps **Crunches—Feet Off Floor** 50 reps **REST ONE MINUTE** **Jackknives** 25 reps **Crunches—Feet Off Floor** 50 reps **REST ONE MINUTE** **Sideways Hyperextensions (Obliques)** 2 sets, each side to failure	**3 SUPER SETS** **Abdominal Wheel** 15–20 reps **Hanging Leg Raises** To failure

Bev Francis

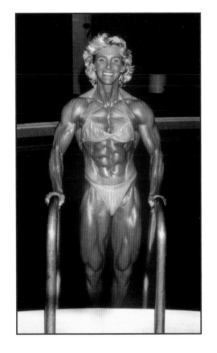

Bev Francis is the most recognizable female body-builder in the world. She has many distinguished accomplishments, including being six-time World Power Lifting Champion and eight-time National Champion who's undefeated in any power-lifting competition. She's a member of the Australian national track-and-field team and a national record holder. She's also an IFBB pro-bodybuilding champion and judge, as well as the star of *Pumping Iron 2*.

Bev is the mother of two and one of the top personal trainers in New York. She's co-owner (with her husband, Steve Weinberger) of the Bev Francis Gold's Gym in Syosset, NY.

"Please note that each exercise is done with no rest between exercises and done to exhaustion/failure," Bev explains. "After all 4 exercises are done, rest one minute and start over. I complete 3–4 giant sets in a workout session."

BEV FRANCIS'S FAVORITE AB ROUTINE (GIANT SET)

EXERCISE	SETS	REPS
Decline Curl-Ups	1	to failure
Reverse Crunch	1	to failure
Hammer Ab Machine	1	to failure
Hanging Knee-Ups	1	to failure

Steve Weinberger

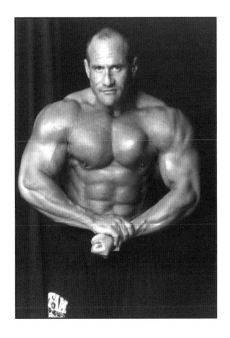

Steve Weinberger is the best bodybuilder and fitness trainer on the scene today. He works with many world-class and professional athletes in all sports and helps anyone he works with achieve their physical best. He's the co-owner of Bev Francis Gold's Gym, which is home to many professional athletes, celebrities, and fitness enthusiasts who want to take advantage of the best-equipped gym in New York. Steve is also the New York City district chairman for the National Physique Committee (NPC), the largest amateur bodybuilding federation in the world. In addition, he's an NPC/IFBB judge and promoter, staging the biggest show in New York—The Bev Francis Atlantic States—which is held to a sold-out crowd every June.

Steve likes to super-set the following routine. "A super set is when you do each exercise consecutively with no rest between them," he elaborates. "I do each exercise to failure, and then after I complete both exercises, I rest for 60 seconds and start again for a total of three sets."

STEVE WEINBERGER'S FAVORITE AB ROUTINE (SUPER SETS)

EXERCISE	SETS	REPS
Rope Crunches	3	to failure
Hanging Knee Raises	3	to failure

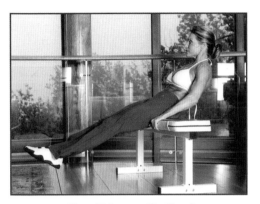

Knee Raises on the Bench

Tosca Reno

Tosca Reno is a fantastic combination of both beauty and brains. This leggy Dutch model has three degrees, speaks four languages, is an accomplished interior designer, and is a veteran writer for *Oxygen* magazine. She's also the author of *The Pan-G Non-Surgical Facelift,* which reveals her secrets to having age-defying skin without going under the knife; while in *The Butt Book,* Tosca gives advice about training the derriere and shares her pro secrets. (Her other book is called *Stretch Marks: Their Cause, Treatment and the Cure.*) The sexy mother of three can also been seen in *MuscleMag International's* latest video, "The Best of MuscleMag."

Tosca loves to train abs and has discovered a few exercises that nail all her muscles in a way that really delivers results. An exercise she calls **"Heels to the Ceiling"** is one of her favorites for isolating the lower abs: Lie on a bench on your back. With legs vertical, toes pointed to the ceiling, contract your abs and push your hips toward the ceiling. Perform 3 or 4 sets of 15–20 reps.

Another exercise is **Knee Raises on the Bench,** which is an excellent exercise for targeting the mid and lower abdominals: Sitting on the edge of a bench and grasping the sides for support, raise your legs out in front of you and contract them in toward your tummy. Repeat this motion for about 20 reps, and do 3–4 sets.

Finally, Tosca performs **Reverse Crunches** lying on a bench, which mainly target the lower waistline. She'll go for 4 sets with 30–50 reps, all of which results in delivering a full abdominal workout.

TOSCA RENO'S FAVORITE AB ROUTINE

EXERCISE	SETS	REPS
Heels to the Ceiling	3–4	15–20
Knee Raises on the Bench	3–4	20
Reverse Crunches	4	30-50

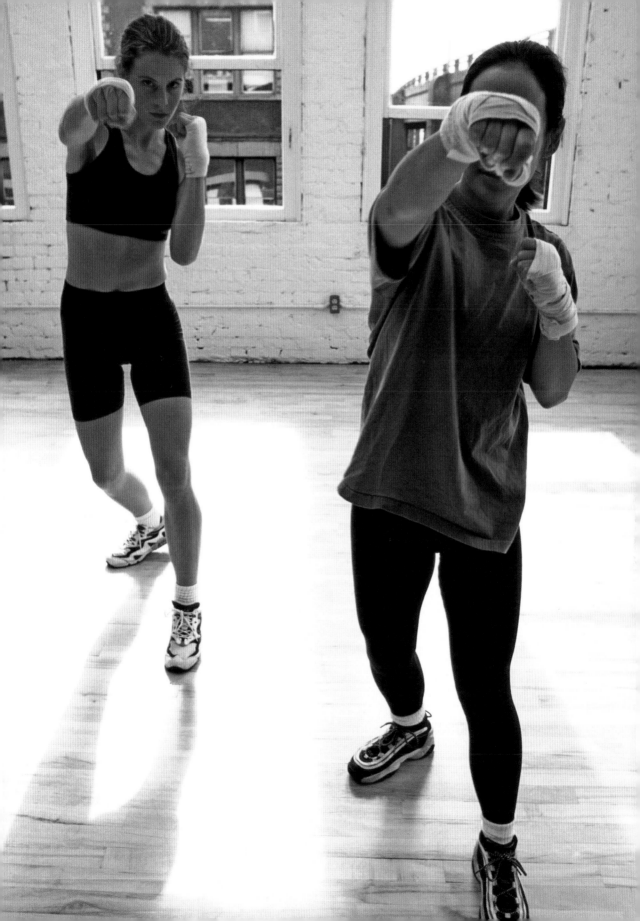

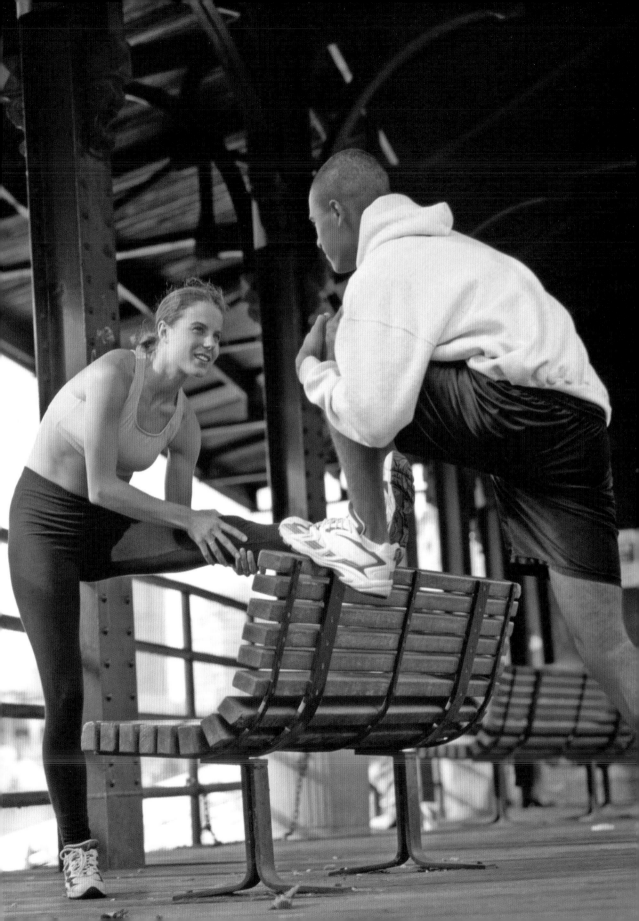

Acknowledgments

It's a great honor and privilege to have the opportunity to relay my knowledge on the subject of abs to you. It's my dream and my mission to help each and every person achieve the body of their dreams, but it would be arrogant and deceitful of me to say that I learned everything about abs on my own. I've been lucky enough to have wonderful teachers who have helped me along the way. If it weren't for all these people, I can honestly say that I wouldn't have half the knowledge I possess about training and nutrition. I'd like to thank you all, and would also like to thank all the people who stood behind me during the good and bad times. I'm blessed to call you all my friends.

The first person I have to acknowledge is the person who is my entire life: my wife, Lisa. It's because of your unconditional love, constant encouragement, and understanding that this book is what it is. Thank you for being so great and for gracing the pages of this book with your beautiful presence. I love you.

I'd also like to thank my mom, Mary, and my dad, Thomas. I couldn't have asked for two better parents. By standing behind me my entire life—whether I was making a good or bad decision—I could always count on unconditional support and love from you both. I'm as proud as a son could be to have you both in my life and to call you Mom and Dad. Thank you both—I love you so much.

In addition, special thanks go to:

Cindy Pearlman—it's always a pleasure to work with you. You did a fantastic job of whipping this book into shape and are a wizard of the written word. Besides being great at what you do, it's your sense of humor that sets you aside from everyone else. I want to thank you for all your contributions and efforts on behalf of this book. I hope that this is just the beginning, and we have many more opportunities to work together in the future.

Hay House—thank you for giving me the opportunity to publish my second work. I specifically want to thank Reid Tracy for giving me the chance to make a positive difference in people's lives with this abdominal book. I'd also like to thank Jill Kramer, Shannon Littrell, Summer McStravick, and Christy Salinas for all your efforts and contributions. You are the people who made this book become a reality through your fantastic editing and beautiful design. Thank you.

Sean Kahlil—we've known each other for 14 years now . . . boy, has time flown! I remember the first time I shot photos with you—whoever would have thought that we'd be working together 14 years later? You've been extremely instrumental in my development as a model by teaching me how to pose correctly and perfect my abilities. I've appeared in more than 200 magazines since we met, so you must have known something! I'd also like to thank you for raising your game once again and shooting the best photos ever seen in a fitness book. And while you can put a price on pictures, you can't put a price on the friendship that we've had and will continue to have. You're definitely in a league of your own.

MET-Rx—it's been an honor and privilege to be associated with such a great company, as your products have played a huge role in the development of my physique and in my everyday eating plan. I'd especially like to thank the following people: Tamara Brown, Kelly Oddo, Marshall Post, Scott Slade, Darren Schneider, Jim Kras, Kristen Kildow, and Robert Walker.

Steve Weinberger—you introduced me to my wife and were best man at my wedding . . . what can I say to you that I haven't already said? You've been like a brother to me, and your advice and teachings have played a huge role in the success I've achieved thus far. I have the utmost respect and admiration for you as a person, and I'm truly thankful to be your friend.

John Edward—it's been well over a year now since we met, and even though I'm supposed to be the one teaching you, I'm learning more from our sessions . . . so who's the teacher now? You've helped me mentally become a better and more rounded person, and we've become great friends. Who would have thought it? The psychic and the fitness trainer. . . . It just goes to show that the mind, body, and spirit all fit together. I'm honored to call you a real friend. (And remember to *put down the cookie!*)

Robert Kennedy—it was your publication, *MuscleMag International,* that started it all for me. Thank you for giving me the opportunity to appear in all your magazines for the past decade. It's because of you that I was able to showcase my talents as a writer, and can now call myself a published author. I can't thank you enough for your advice, wisdom, and friendship. Thank you for all the publicity you've given to me over the years—you're a good friend and a man of your word.

Kerri-Lee Brown—thank you for giving me the opportunity to write my first feature article in *American Health & Fitness.* You've been a great friend in this business. May you and Craig have many, many years of happiness, and may your magazine continue to prosper.

ESPN2's *Cold Pizza*—I just want to thank everyone down at the show for giving me a shot at working on television and making me feel so welcome. Thank you Denise Cavannaugh, Mechell E. Harris, Jay Crawford, Leslie Maxie, Thea Andrews, Kit Hoover, and Zach Lebowitz.

Richard Perez Feria—we started this journey together, and although we didn't finish it together, I'm still aware of the fact that if it weren't for you I wouldn't be at this point in my life. I'd just like to say thank you for continuing to be a very good friend, along with congratulations on becoming the editor of *People en Español.* Lisa and I are extremely proud of such a huge accomplishment—continued success from your two Long Island friends.

Larry Pepe—your expertise and practical knowledge in the fields of psychology, motivation, and nutrition have been invaluable. You have my endorsement now and in the future as one of the most knowledgeable mental and physical teachers, and I look forward to a lifetime of friendship. Thanks.

Scott Connelly—even though we've been out of touch the last couple years, I still consider you a friend. It was you who was responsible for bringing me to MET-Rx, and it was you who taught me a great deal about nutrition and supplementation. Being able to learn from someone whom I consider one of the smartest men on the planet was definitely my privilege. Thank you, and I wish you the best of health and success in the future.

Jimmy "The Bull" Pellechia—we've worked together for close to a decade and have traveled all over this country together numerous times. The adventures we've had and the stories we could tell would fill ten books. Without a doubt, you're one of a kind, and I'm proud to call you my friend.

Now I want to thank the following families for your love and encouragement. I appreciate it a great deal—thank you:

The Sepe family—Thomas, Mary, Thomas, Susan, Laci, Uncle Joe, Aunt Cathy, Dianne, Anthony, and Gina.

The Pelcher family—thank you Rich, Robin, Isabelle, and Matthew.

The Grunewald family—thank you, Thomas, Pat, and Danny, for your kindness and support.

The Terry family—Karen, Bob, Bobby, Shawn, Nicole, and Rachel.

Thomas Sepe—you've led your life by great example. Not only are you hardworking, but you're a good husband and father. You're also a great brother who's never not answered the call when I needed you, *and* I'm lucky to have you as my friend, too.

Scott Pryhocki—our friendship has stood the test of time, and we've been through a lot together. Who would have thought that we'd both turn out the way we did? Those who know us say we're exactly the same . . . well, I take that as a compliment.

I'd like to thank all those who contributed to this book in one form or another:

Bev Francis Gold's Gym—I couldn't think of a better place to shoot these workout photos. Also, if I had to choose only one gym in the world for my own training, this would be the one. Thank you to all my friends for your support and friendships.

Richard Jankura—your enthusiasm and positive attitude toward this book made life on all the photo sets a much less stressful atmosphere. Thank you for helping with the shoots. You've proven time and time again that you're a great friend, as well as a person who can be counted on.

StrengthNet Models—Adam Silver, thank you for providing us with most of our fitness models. (**Stengthnet.com** is a great place to find fitness models.) Thanks to the models for brightening up the pages of my book. Nice job to Paige Grofe, Brienne Michelle, Peter Gaeth, Stuart Miller, and David August. I'd also like to thank my friends and models Davana Medina, Anthony Catanzaro, and Jane Awad; and give a special thanks to Jason Fabini, Bev Francis, K.C. Armstrong, Leslie Maxie, Mike Ruiz, and Derek Panza.

Theresa Hartle—thank you for looking out for my best interests and being such a great friend. Your advice and tireless efforts on behalf of both books is greatly appreciated.

PMK-HBH—thank you Jill Fritzo, Jen Plante, and Jon Streep for all your hard work.

Marc Chamlin—thanks for all your advice. It's been very helpful.

GNC—Charlie Chiverini, thanks for all your efforts on behalf of the book.

NPC—the National Physique Committee is the best bodybuilding federation in the world, and I'm proud to be a judge and promoter for the organization. Thank you for all your help and support over the years. I'd especially like to thank Jim Manion—I have a tremendous amount of respect for your tireless efforts on behalf of the NPC.

Joseph Gazio—I was a teenager who thought he knew everything when I walked into the gym for the first time. It was you who took the time to show me how to do the exercises properly and encouraged me to pursue my body's full potential. Thanks for taking the time to help me out. I've never forgotten, and I will always remember.

Tony Pandolfo—how many 60-year-old guys can wear a tank top and turn the heads of girls who are 30 years younger? Your physique has stood the test of time and is a testament to the fact that you practice what you preach. Thanks for teaching me so much about bodybuilding and nutrition.

And finally, thanks to the fans who have purchased my second book. Get ready for number three.

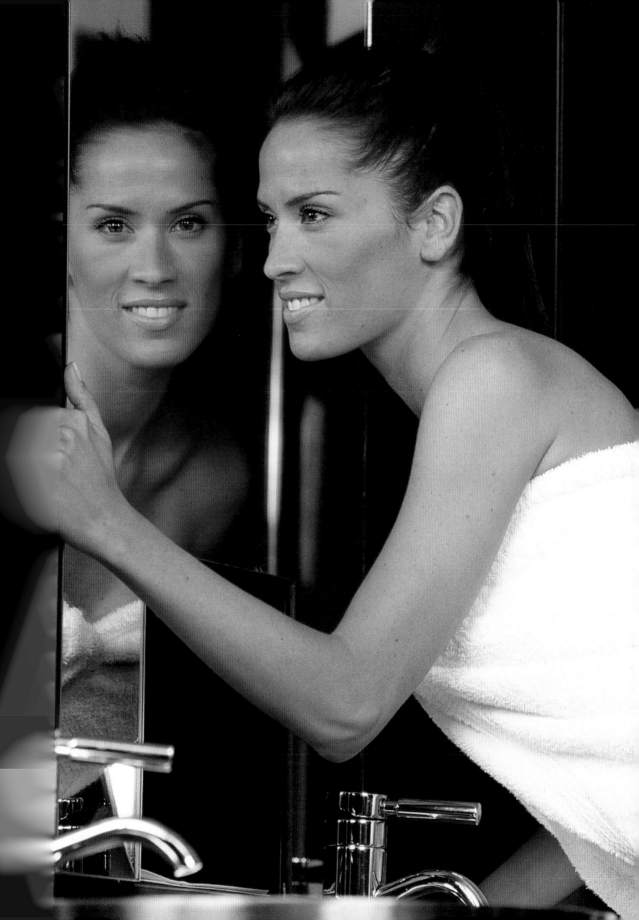

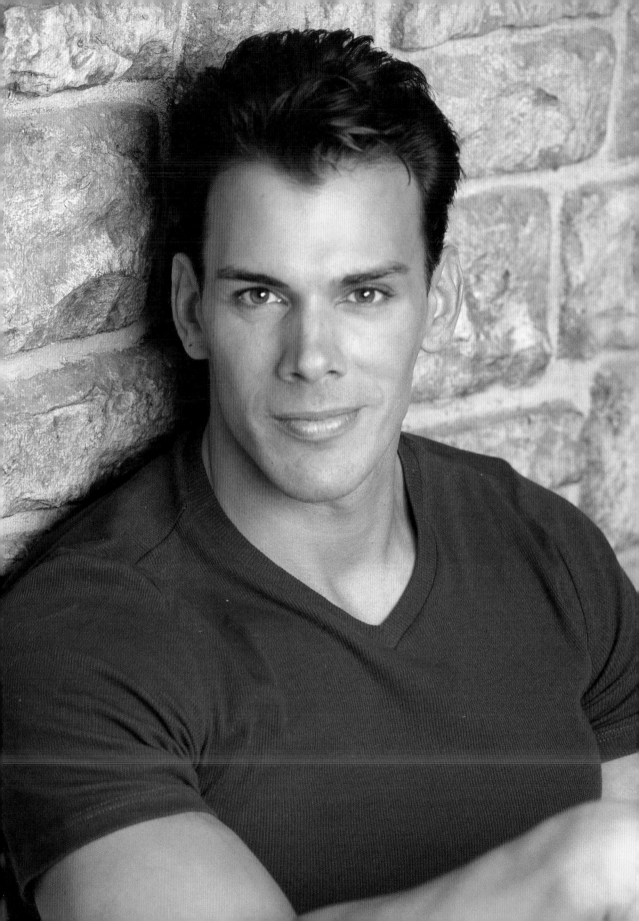

About the Author

To distill **Frank Sepe** in brief isn't as easy as one may think. Sure, as one of the most photographed physique models of all time, Frank has graced hundreds of fitness magazine covers (*Muscle and Fitness, MuscleMag International, Iron Man, Muscular Development,* and *American Health & Fitness,* to name a few), romance-book jackets, and fitness encyclopedias; and he's been the subject of some 500 fan Websites. But this isn't nearly the full picture . . . not by a long shot.

Frank is the resident fitness expert for ESPN2's show *Cold Pizza.* He's also a highly respected writer who's the author of *THE TRUTH: The Only Fitness Book You'll Ever Need,* and a contributing editor and monthly columnist for leading magazines (*MuscleMag International, American Health & Fitness*); a consultant/fitness source for dozens of TV, news, and radio shows; as well as for the *Oxygen, Cosmopolitan,* and *American Curves* women's-fitness publications.

He's also a working actor *(The Devil and Daniel Webster, Carlito's Way)* who's made frequent TV guest appearances *(Live with Regis and Kelly, The Howard Stern Show, Late Night with Conan O'Brien, The Rick Sanchez Show).* He also maintains private personal-training clients (including celebrities and professional athletes) and a full schedule as a spokesperson for fitness giant MET-Rx—all while promoting accredited physique programs. To contact Frank, please e-mail: **mail@franksepe.com**.

We hope you enjoyed this Hay House book.
If you'd like to receive a free catalog featuring additional
Hay House books and products, or if you'd like information
about the Hay Foundation, please contact:

Hay House, Inc.
P.O. Box 5100
Carlsbad, CA 92018-5100

(760) 431-7695 or **(800) 654-5126**
(760) 431-6948 (fax) or **(800) 650-5115 (fax)**
www.hayhouse.com

———

Published and distributed in Australia by:
Hay House Australia Pty. Ltd. • 18/36 Ralph St. • Alexandria NSW 2015 •
Phone: 612-9669-4299 • *Fax:* 612-9669-4144 • www.hayhouse.com.au

Published and distributed in the United Kingdom by:
Hay House UK, Ltd. • Unit 62, Canalot Studios •
222 Kensal Rd., London W10 5BN • *Phone:* 44-20-8962-1230 •
Fax: 44-20-8962-1239 • www.hayhouse.co.uk

Published and distributed in the Republic of South Africa by:
Hay House SA (Pty), Ltd., P.O. Box 990, Witkoppen 2068 •
Phone/Fax: 2711-7012233 • orders@psdprom.co.za

Distributed in Canada by:
Raincoast • 9050 Shaughnessy St., Vancouver, B.C. V6P 6E5 •
Phone: (604) 323-7100 • *Fax:* (604) 323-2600

———

Sign up via the Hay House USA Website to receive the Hay House online
newsletter and stay informed about what's going on with your favorite authors.
You'll receive bimonthly announcements about: Discounts and Offers,
Special Events, Product Highlights, Free Excerpts, Giveaways, and more!
www.hayhouse.com